Sonoanatomy for Anaesthetists

Sonoanatomy for Anaesthetists

Edward Lin
Consultant in Pain Management and Anaesthesia,
Glenfield Hospital, University of Leicester Hospitals
NHS Trust, Leicester, UK

Atul Gaur
Consultant Anaesthetist, Glenfield Hospital,
University of Leicester Hospitals NHS Trust,
Leicester, UK

Michael Jones
Consultant Anaesthetist, Glenfield Hospital,
University of Leicester Hospitals NHS Trust,
Leicester, UK

Aamer Ahmed
Consultant Anaesthetist, Glenfield Hospital,
University of Leicester Hospitals NHS Trust,
Leicester, UK

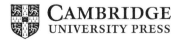

CAMBRIDGE
UNIVERSITY PRESS

CAMBRIDGE
UNIVERSITY PRESS

University Printing House, Cambridge CB2 8BS, United Kingdom

Published in the United States of America by Cambridge University Press,
New York

Cambridge University Press is part of the University of Cambridge.

It furthers the University's mission by disseminating knowledge in the
pursuit of education, learning and research at the highest international
levels of excellence.

www.cambridge.org
Information on this title: www.cambridge.org/9780521106665

© E. Lin, M. Jones, A. Gaur and A. Ahmed 2012
Artwork created by Emily Evans, © Cambridge University Press

First published 2012
4th printing 2016

Printed in the United Kingdom by Bell & Bain Ltd, Glasgow

A catalogue record for this publication is available from the British Library

Library of Congress Cataloging-in-Publication Data

Sonoanatomy for anesthetists / Edward Lin ... [et al.].
    p.   cm.
ISBN 978 0 521 10666 5 (Paperback)
I. Lin, Ted, 1945–
   [DNLM: 1. Anatomy, Cross-Sectional.   2. Ultrasonography –
methods.   3. Anaesthesia – methods. WN 208]
616.07′543–dc23   2011049738

ISBN 978 0 521 10666 5 Paperback

CONTENTS

PREFACE

The introduction of ultrasound into the clinical practice of anaesthetists and pain specialists brings potentially great benefit to clinicians and their patients. The ability to visualise what lies beneath the surface while performing nerve blocks, cannulations and injections has rekindled an increasing awareness of the need for a thorough understanding of regional anatomy and its relation to ultrasound, if the patterns in ultrasound scans are to be confidently interpreted.

This book aims to help its readers to identify the anatomy revealed in an ultrasound scan – the sonoanatomy. In order to achieve this, clinicians need to draw on their surface anatomy, their experience with landmark techniques and their knowledge of regional anatomy, whilst improving their skills with the ultrasound machine.

The authors have tried to illustrate some of the basic relationships between surface anatomy, regional anatomy and the ultrasound scans for most of the common interventions performed by anaesthetists and pain medicine clinicians. The book does not aim to provide step-by-step recipes for individual procedures, which are continually evolving and changing. Rather, it tries to present some basic guidelines which will enable readers to develop their own approaches to interventions.

This volume is intended to be a practical book, not just to be read and placed on a shelf, but hopefully one that will be taken into the workplace and used as an aid during clinical practice.

Getting the best scan

Choosing a probe

Select the most appropriate probe for the particular scan required. Probes vary in their:

- operating frequency range – higher ultrasound frequencies provide better discrimination of fine detail but have lower penetration because of increased attenuation by the tissues.
- physical size – the smaller the probe, the smaller its 'footprint' when placed on the patient.
- the width of the tissue field scanned – an ultrasound probe scans a 'slice' of tissue approximately 1–3 mm thick, with a width dependent on the size of the probe.

Common types of probe available (Fig. 1) are:

Linear   These probes have a flat face and give a parallel-sided scan field approximately 1 mm 'thick'. Linear probes operate at frequencies typically between 5 and 18 MHz. They come in different widths, between 20 and 40 mm, with correspondingly different lengths of probe footprint. These are the best general-purpose probes.

Hockey-stick   These are small probes that can be held with a 'fountain-pen' grip. They are appropriate for small or paediatric patients. They are also useful for awkward areas such as close to the clavicle or posterior to the medial malleolus, where the physical size of the wider probes may make it difficult to manipulate the probe or obtain good skin contact. The less the width of the probe, the smaller its footprint, but the narrower the field covered in the scan and the more difficult it is to identify the anatomy in the scan.

Curvilinear   These probes have a curved face giving a fan-shaped scan field. The field is diverging, with

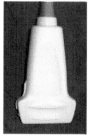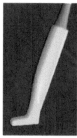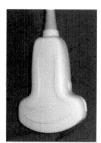

Linear probe   Hockey-stick probe   Curvilinear probe

Fig 1 Three common types of ultrasound probe

curvilinear distortion in the horizontal direction – analogous to that seen with a fish-eye lens in photography. A more panoramic view is therefore obtained in the scan, which can make identification of the local anatomy easier. Curvilinear probes generally operate at relatively lower frequencies (typically 2–5 MHz), giving greater depths of penetration but with coarser discrimination.

Choosing the frequency

The frequency of ultrasound can significantly alter the appearance of the scan obtained. The frequency will determine both the depth of penetration and the discrimination of detail in the scan. Unfortunately there is a trade-off between depth of penetration and discrimination of detail. The higher the frequency the better the resolution of detail in the scan, but the lower the penetration of tissues. Typically a linear probe operating at 10 MHz gives good resolution of detail but only provides good penetration to depths of 2–3 cm. Targets beyond this range are more difficult to visualize (Fig. 2).

A curvilinear probe working at 2–5 MHz can penetrate soft tissues reasonably well up to 4–10 cm, but the discrimination of detail is coarser (Fig. 3).

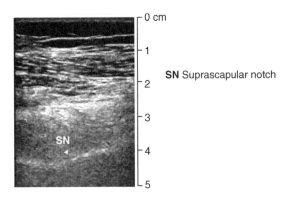

SN Suprascapular notch

Fig 2 **High resolution but low penetration:**
a high-resolution scan of the suprascapular notch,
using a linear probe at 10 MHz

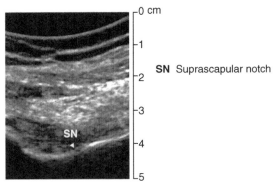

SN Suprascapular notch

Fig 3 **High penetration but low resolution: a low-resolution**
scan of the suprascapular notch, using a curvilinear probe
at 4 MHz

Gain control

This control is equivalent to the 'brightness' control, and it may make targets easier to see in the scan (Fig. 4). It changes the overall appearance of the scan from dark (black) to bright (white). It will not necessarily make targets easier to distinguish or identify. More sophisticated machines can increase the gain at a selected depth, known as time gain compensation (TGC). This feature can be useful when trying to visualize more distal targets at depths where the penetration of the ultrasound is poor.

Depth

Use the depth control to place the target area at approximately two-thirds of the total depth of the scan.

Focus

Some machines have a focus control which enhances image quality at a chosen level. This should be set just deep to the target area.

Identifying the anatomy in a scan

Gross anatomy

Orientation in an ultrasound scan is predominantly a process of pattern recognition. Knowledge of the anatomy in the region being scanned is essential in interpreting and identifying structures in the scan. Using the surface anatomy to aid accurate and consistent placement of the probe helps to obtain a scan with a familiar pattern.

(A)

(B)

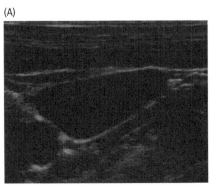
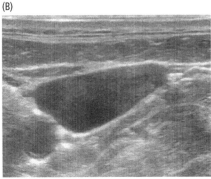

Fig 4 **A scan of the carotid artery and internal jugular vein: (A) with the gain adjusted too low; (B) with the scan gain increased**

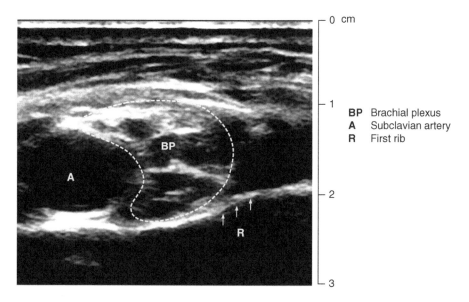

BP Brachial plexus
A   Subclavian artery
R   First rib

Fig 5 **Vascular and bony landmarks in an ultrasound scan: locating the brachial plexus**

Scan landmarks

Use vascular and bony landmarks to orientate in a scan. For example, use the subclavian artery and first rib to orientate in a supraclavicular scan of the brachial plexus (Fig. 5).

Tracking

In some patients it may prove difficult to identify a target structure in a scan with the probe at a particular location. This can often be solved by identifying the structure at an alternative location where it is easy to see, and then 'tracking' it back to the desired location.

For example, if it is proving difficult to find the ulnar nerve at mid forearm level, first find the nerve at the wrist, where it can easily be located between the ulnar artery and the flexor carpi ulnaris tendon. Then 'track' it proximally to forearm level by slowly sliding the probe up the forearm while taking care to keep the ulnar nerve in view (Fig. 6). As the nerve and artery are tracked proximally it can be seen that although the nerve starts adjacent to the artery in the wrist its course diverges from the artery in the proximal forearm, where it can be blocked with reduced risk of arterial puncture.

Anisotropy

Slight adjustments of the probe about its long axis (tilting the probe) when at the scan position can greatly improve the view of a target or even reveal its presence when previously unseen (Fig. 7). This is a result of altering the angle at which the ultrasound waves strike the target and thus optimizing the reflections received by the probe. This effect is referred to as *anisotropy*.

Fig. 8 compares two views of the median nerve obtained with the probe in exactly the same position on the forearm. The only difference between the two scans is a slight change of the probe angle about its long axis, to maximize and minimize the anisotropic effect.

Recognizing different tissues in an ultrasound scan

The use of ultrasound when scanning body tissues demonstrates some differences between tissues. Detail in the scans is dependent on the wavelength, which is inversely dependent on frequency. The production of targets (bright reflections) in a scan relies on reflection of ultrasound, the reflected waves having to pass back to the probe in order to be

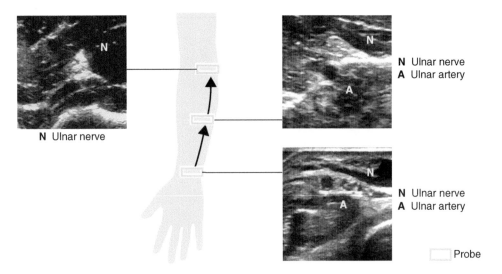

N Ulnar nerve

N Ulnar nerve
A Ulnar artery

N Ulnar nerve
A Ulnar artery

☐ Probe

Fig 6 Tracking the ulnar nerve from wrist to forearm

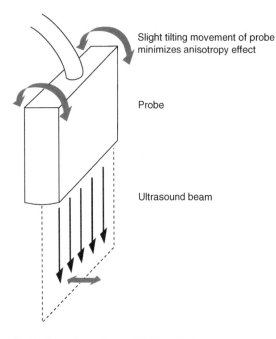

Slight tilting movement of probe minimizes anisotropy effect

Probe

Ultrasound beam

Fig 7 Tilting the probe to minimize anisotropy

received. This means that the visibility of a target relies on reflection and can be attenuated by scattering. Reflection at a boundary between different tissues is determined by the differences in acoustic impedances of the tissues.

The best-defined targets have boundaries (surfaces) which separate media with the greatest mismatch of acoustic impedances – for example, between soft tissue and air, soft tissue and bone, soft tissue and fluid. Some representative acoustic impedances are shown in Table 1.

Modern machines have tissue harmonic imaging, which uses harmonics of the ultrasound beam to reduce the effects of scattering and improve tissue resolution.

Nerves

Peripheral nerves have a granular appearance in cross-section due to the echogenicity of the endoneurium tissue around the nerve fascicles (Fig. 9). They appear less echogenic when viewed more centrally. In longitudinal section the fascicles are visible as parallel streaks within the nerve.

Tendons

Tendons may easily be confused with nerves, but usually the granularity in cross-section and the streaking in longitudinal section are finer, and the appearance is more homogeneous (Fig. 10). Distinguish between nerves and tendons in a scan by tracking. Track nerves from areas where they are

(A)

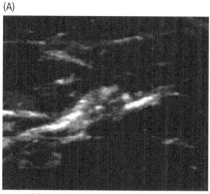

(B)

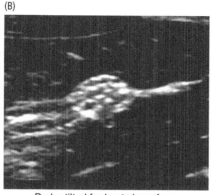

Fig 8 Two views of the
median nerve: (A) poor and
(B) good probe adjustment
to reduce anisotropy effect

View with poor probe adjustment

Probe tilted for best view of nerve

Fig 8 Two views of the median nerve: (A) poor and (B) good probe adjustment to reduce anisotropy effect

more easily identifiable, or track tendons to the muscles they are attached to. Alternatively, ask the patient to make appropriate movements, which cause the tendons to move in the scan while the nerves remain relatively stationary.

Muscle

Muscle is coarsely speckled in cross-section, with more dense connective tissue outlining the fascicles.

Table 1 **Values of acoustic impedance for different tissues**

Tissue	Velocity of sound (m s^{-1})	Acoustic impedance (kg m^{-2} s^{-1}) $\times 10^{-6}$
Gas	330	0.0004
Fat	1470	1.43
Blood	1570	1.53
Muscle	1568	1.63
Bone	4080	6.12

In longitudinal section the fascicles produce coarse irregular striations (Fig. 11).

Bone

Bone can only be visualized in a scan by the proximal surface that is exposed to the incident ultrasound. Since the ultrasound waves do not penetrate this proximal boundary (as they do in the case of soft tissue structures such as blood vessels and nerves), the proximal surface of a bone in the scan leaves a dark region or 'drop-out shadow' distally.

Therefore bones do not appear in an ultrasound scan as a two-dimensional structure or cross-section. Instead, bones are recognized as hyperechoic (bright) profiles proximal to a dark drop-out shadow (Fig. 12).

(A)

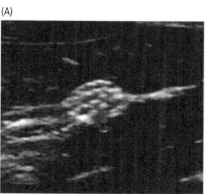

(B)

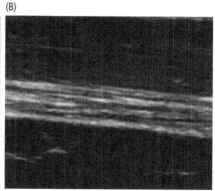

Fig 9 **Ultrasound appearance of nerve – fascicular pattern**

Cross-section of nerve

Longitudinal section of nerve

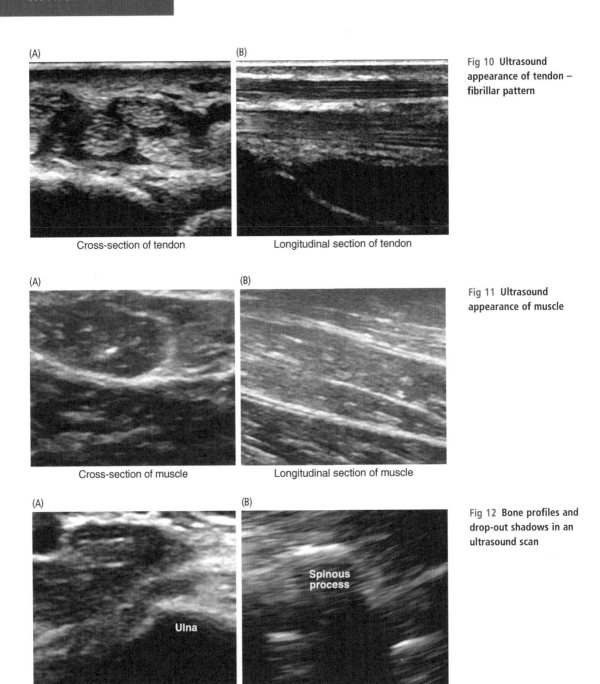

(A)   (B)

Cross-section of tendon   Longitudinal section of tendon

Fig 10 Ultrasound appearance of tendon – fibrillar pattern

(A)   (B)

Cross-section of muscle   Longitudinal section of muscle

Fig 11 Ultrasound appearance of muscle

(A)   (B)

Spinous process

Ulna

Ulnar shadow at the wrist   Shadow of lumbar spinous process

Fig 12 Bone profiles and drop-out shadows in an ultrasound scan

Blood vessels

Arteries and veins are readily recognized because of the low echogenicity of the blood they contain. Arteries retain their circular cross-section and pulsate even when pressure is applied to the probe, unlike accompanying veins, which are of greater cross-sectional area but with a more irregular cross-section and a tendency to collapse when pressure is applied to the probe (Fig. 13). Occasionally a valve may be seen in the lumen of a large central vein as a pulsatile intraluminal echo.

(A)

(B)

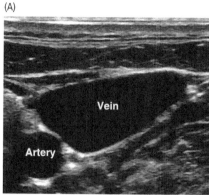
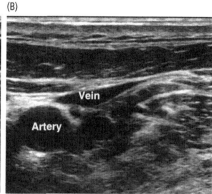

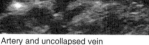

Fig 13 **Scans of an artery and a vein, showing collapse of vein with pressure applied to probe**

Artery and uncollapsed vein

Artery and collapsed vein due to probe pressue

Post-cystic enhancement

Often a bright area can be seen distal to a fluid-filled cyst or vessel (Fig. 14). This is the combined result of (1) low attenuation of ultrasound waves as they pass through the vessel, (2) refraction and (3) 'edge shadows'. The edge shadows are caused by scattering of the incident ultrasound waves from the edges of the vessel.

Uses of ultrasound in procedures

Guiding the needle in regional anaesthesia

Use of ultrasound enables real-time guidance of the needle in regional anaesthesia. The ultrasound beam is only approximately 1 mm in thickness. In order to guide the needle it is necessary to obtain the best possible view of the needle and needle tip.

Obtaining a good view of the needle

A good view of the needle in the scan requires the needle to be in the plane of the ultrasound beam. In addition, the angle between the needle and the face of the probe should be as small as possible in order to maximize the reflection of ultrasound waves back to the probe (Fig. 15). When the angle between the needle and probe face is greater than 45 degrees poor visibility of the needle results, since the ultrasound is reflected from the needle at an angle rather than back to the probe (high-visibility needles can improve this poor visibility).

Ideally, try to maintain an angle of less than 30 degrees between needle and probe face. The best view of the needle is obtained when the needle is parallel to the face of the probe. Keeping the bevel of the needle tip facing the probe improves needle tip visualization.

In-plane and out-of-plane needling techniques

In-plane needling refers to needle insertion parallel to the ultrasound beam, keeping the needle within the plane of the beam, so that the length of the needle and its tip are visualized during insertion. Out-of-plane needle insertion is performed with the needle perpendicular to the ultrasound beam. In this case the needle is only visualized as a hyperechoic spot where it crosses the plane of the ultrasound beam.

In-plane needling As long as the whole needle, and in particular its tip, lies in the plane of the ultrasound beam, it can be observed as it passes along its track, and puncturing unwanted structures such as blood vessels and pleura can be avoided (Fig. 16A). However, because the ultrasound beam is only 1–3 mm thick, it is easy to only obtain a partial view of the needle, leaving the tip invisible because it is out of the plane of the ultrasound beam (Fig. 16B). In such a case the puncture of unwanted structures is more likely. Therefore in-plane needling is the safest technique to use, provided good alignment of the needle is maintained.

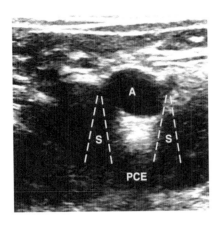

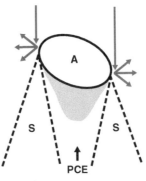

Incident ultrasound scattered from edges of artery

Fig 14 Post-cystic enhancement

A   Artery
PCE Post-cystic enhancement
S   Edge shadows

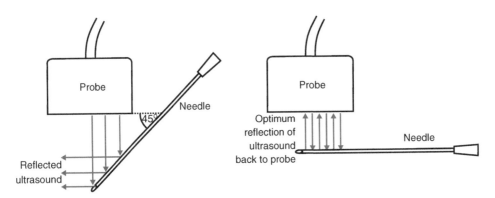

Fig 15 **The effect of different angles between needle and probe: poor visibility with a steep angle; good visibility when the needle is parallel to the probe**

Out-of-plane needling Often gives an advantage in identifying surrounding anatomy but does increase the risks of puncturing unwanted structures, since the needle tip is out of plane and not visible. A hyperechoic 'dot' in the scan marks the point at which the needle crosses the plane of the ultrasound beam. The position of the needle tip can be located by sliding the probe along the needle axis until this hyperechoic dot disappears. In this position, tilting the probe about its long axis causes the needle tip to appear and disappear, confirming its position in the ultrasound beam. Out-of-plane needling may be used for practical reasons such as passing a catheter for continuous infusion blockade. In such a case the catheter needs to be inserted parallel to a nerve, and needling out of plane can make this significantly easier (Fig. 17). The track of the needle in out-of-plane needling is observed indirectly on an ultrasound scan by looking for the movement of tissue in the scan caused by the passage of the needle.

Observation of local anaesthetic spread

When performing regional anaesthetic blocks, the distribution or spread of the injected local anaesthetic can determine whether or not an

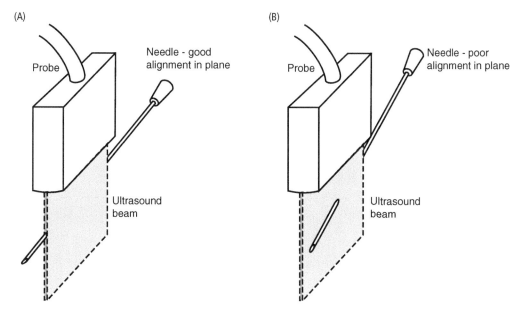

Fig 16 In-plane needling with (A) good and (B) poor alignment (needle tip out of plane)

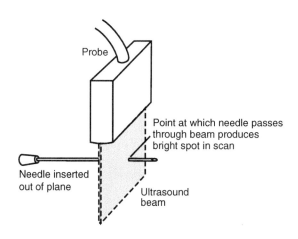

Fig 17 Out-of-plane needling

effective block is obtained. Thus when using ultrasound guidance for regional anaesthesia it is useful to observe the spread of local anaesthetic as it is injected.

Fig. 18 shows how the local anaesthetic in a femoral nerve block can spread away from the nerve (B) rather than around the nerve (A). This might occur even in the presence of good muscle twitches if a nerve stimulator is used.

Good spread of local anaesthetic in a regional block can be observed in real time as the local anaesthetic, which is echolucent, can be seen to surround the target nerves as injection takes place.

Fig. 19 shows an ultrasound scan of the supraclavicular brachial plexus, with local anaesthetic surrounding the trunks of the plexus.

Checking perineural catheter placement

Insertion of a perineural catheter can be used in cases where continuous infusion blockade is required (Fig. 20). Insertion of a catheter to lie alongside the nerve being blocked can sometimes be difficult, as the track of the catheter may not stay close to the nerve. Needling out of plane can facilitate passing the catheter. The final catheter position can be checked using ultrasound, but the catheter usually appears only intermittently as bright dots in the scan. Injection of a small quantity of air under ultrasound observation can also help confirm placement.

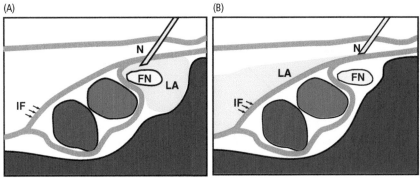

(A) (B)

Fig 18 (A) Good spread and (B) poor spread of local anaesthetic in a femoral nerve block, depending on whether the needle penetrates the iliopectineal fascia

LA Local anaesthetic
FN Femoral nerve
N Needle
IF Iliopectineal fascia

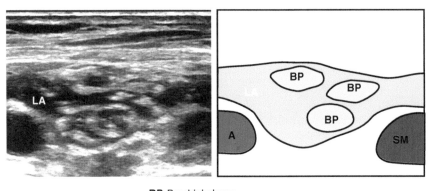

Fig 19 Spread of local anaesthetic in brachial plexus block, showing local anaesthetic surrounding the divisions of the plexus

BP Brachial plexus
LA Local anaesthetic
A Subclavian artery
SM Scalenus medius muscle

Guiding intravascular cannulation

Intravascular cannulation can be guided by ultrasound, either for central venous cannulation or for peripheral vessel cannulation in cases where peripheral vessels are not easily visualized.

Ultrasound can be used to detect an appropriate vessel, check entry of a guide wire into the vessel and check final placement of the cannula into the vessel. Fig. 21 shows the stages in cannulation of an internal jugular vein, using an in-plane technique.

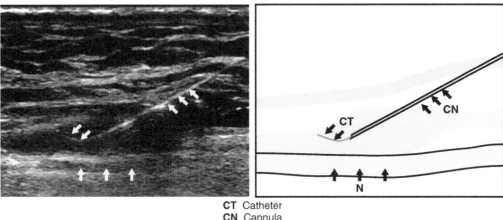

CT Catheter
CN Cannula
N Nerve

Fig 20 **Perineural catheter placement with cannula**

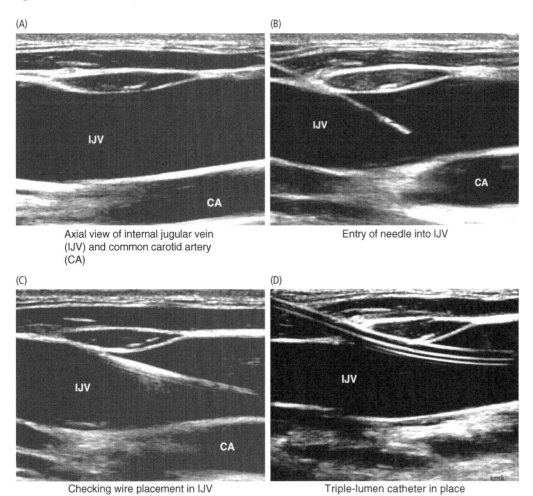

(A) Axial view of internal jugular vein (IJV) and common carotid artery (CA)

(B) Entry of needle into IJV

(C) Checking wire placement in IJV

(D) Triple-lumen catheter in place

Fig 21 **Four stages in the cannulation of an internal jugular vein**

Anatomy of the suprascapular nerve

The suprascapular nerve (SSN) is a mixed motor and sensory nerve which originates from (C4), C5, C6. It passes across the upper part of the posterior triangle of the neck and through the suprascapular notch under the suprascapular ligament, while the accompanying suprascapular artery passes over the suprascapular ligament. The SSN innervates the supraspinatus and infraspinatus muscles, as well as being the sensory supply to the glenohumeral joint. It is often blocked to relieve chronic shoulder pain. Fig. 1.1 is a view of the scapula from above, showing the supraspinatus fossa.

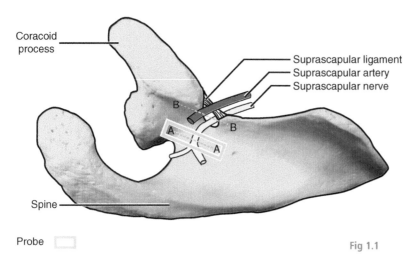

Fig 1.1

Probe placement for suprascapular nerve block

With the patient in a sitting position, apply a curvilinear probe just medial to the acromioclavicular joint and parallel to the scapular spine. The probe should be placed with its face above and parallel to the spine of the scapula. Start with the beam directed caudally onto the floor of the supraspinatus fossa (line AA in Fig. 1.1), and scan forwards by tilting the probe until the beam reaches the anterior wall of the fossa (line BB in Fig. 1.1), where the suprascapular notch comes into view.

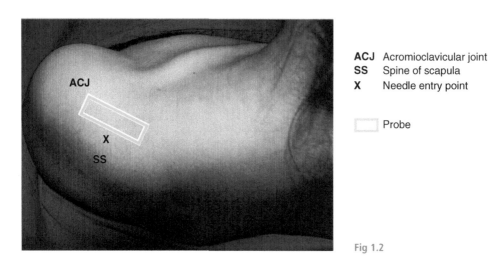

ACJ   Acromioclavicular joint
SS   Spine of scapula
X   Needle entry point

Probe

Fig 1.2

Scan of suprascapular notch

When the plane of the ultrasound beam lies along the more dorsal line (AA in Fig. 1.1), the floor of the supraspinatus fossa is visible as a continuous bony profile. As the ultrasound plane is swept anteriorly by tilting the probe, the suprascapular notch appears as a break or step in this profile. Sometimes the suprascapular artery is visible on the scan, usually lateral to and above the nerve. The nerve itself is not usually seen.

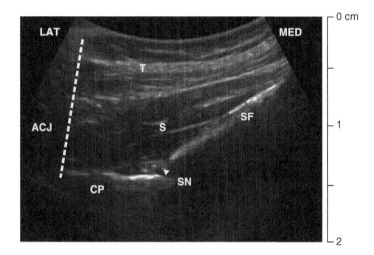

CP	Coracoid process
SF	Floor of supraspinatus fossa
T	Trapezius muscle
S	Supraspinatus muscle
SN	Suprascapular notch
ACJ	Drop-out shadow from acromioclavicular joint

Fig 1.3

Diagram of scan

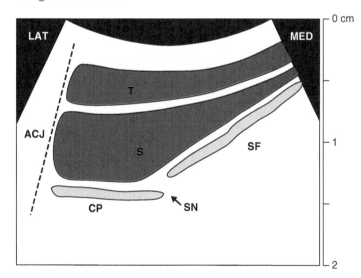

CP	Coracoid process
SF	Floor of supraspinatus fossa
T	Trapezius muscle
S	Supraspinatus muscle
SN	Suprascapular notch
ACJ	Drop-out shadow from acromioclavicular joint

Fig 1.4

Tips and complications Prescan to obtain the best view of the suprascapular notch, and mark the position of the probe before skin preparation and needle puncture. Confirm proximity of the needle tip to the suprascapular nerve by using a nerve stimulator set to 0.5–1 mA and observing twitching of supraspinatus fibres in the scan. Insert the needle out of plane, aiming for the centre of the suprascapular notch. By 'walking' the needle anteriorly it is possible to enter the notch. Take care not to pass the needle through the notch too far, in case of pleural puncture.

Anatomy of the supraclavicular brachial plexus

The brachial plexus is formed from the spinal roots C5–T1, which combine to form superior, middle and inferior trunks in the neck. These trunks emerge into the posterior triangle of the neck, together with the subclavian artery, from the space between the anterior and middle scalene muscles. They can be found lying superficially (1–2 cm deep) in the base of the posterior triangle. The trunks then pass across the upper surface of the first rib, where they lie posterior and lateral to the artery, which in turn lies posterior to the vein. The trunks exit the supraclavicular region by passing beneath the clavicle, where they divide into anterior and posterior divisions behind the clavicle.

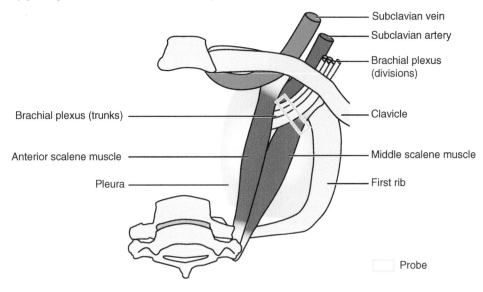

Fig 2.1

Probe placement for supraclavicular brachial plexus block

Identify the sides of the posterior triangle of the neck. The anterior side is the posterior border of sternocleidomastoid, the posterior side is the anterior border of trapezius, and the base is the clavicle. A linear probe is applied across the base of the posterior triangle. Keep the plane of the beam pointing in a caudal direction parallel to the longitudinal axis of the body, so that the beam cuts across the brachial plexus and artery as they lie on the first rib.

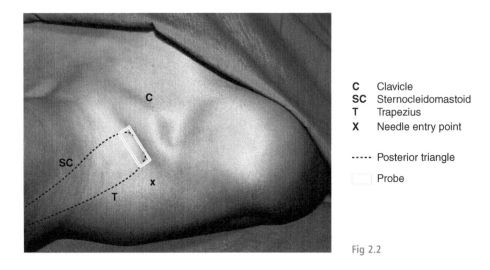

C   Clavicle
SC   Sternocleidomastoid
T   Trapezius
X   Needle entry point

----- Posterior triangle
Probe

Fig 2.2

Scan of supraclavicular brachial plexus

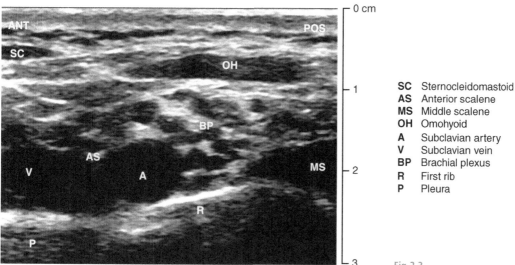

SC	Sternocleidomastoid
AS	Anterior scalene
MS	Middle scalene
OH	Omohyoid
A	Subclavian artery
V	Subclavian vein
BP	Brachial plexus
R	First rib
P	Pleura

Fig 2.3

Diagram of scan

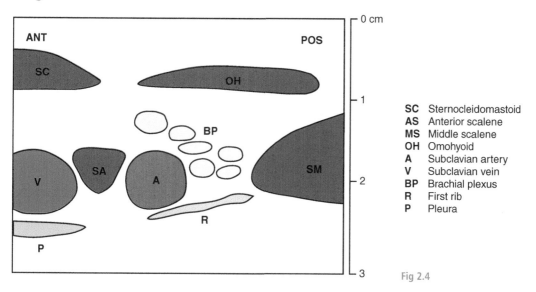

SC	Sternocleidomastoid
AS	Anterior scalene
MS	Middle scalene
OH	Omohyoid
A	Subclavian artery
V	Subclavian vein
BP	Brachial plexus
R	First rib
P	Pleura

Fig 2.4

Tips and complications Insert the needle from the posterior edge of the probe in plane, keeping the tip in view, and keep the plane of the ultrasound beam over the rib. Maintain a shallow trajectory of the needle by removing the patient's pillow from the side to be blocked or by using a head ring, as the brachial plexus is superficial in this position. These precautions reduce the risk of inadvertent pleural puncture.

Depositing local anaesthetic in the 'corner pocket' between the subclavian artery and the first rib pushes the brachial plexus up and away from the rib, and ensures coverage of the inferior trunk and divisions.

Complications include pneumothorax and puncture of subclavian vessels or the thyrocervical trunk, which may cross the trajectory of the needle to the brachial plexus. The phrenic nerve lies on the anterior surface of the anterior scalene muscle and is often blocked as well as the brachial plexus.

Anatomy of the interscalene brachial plexus

In the posterior triangle of the neck, the roots of the brachial plexus (C5–T1) can be found in the space between the anterior and middle scalene muscles.

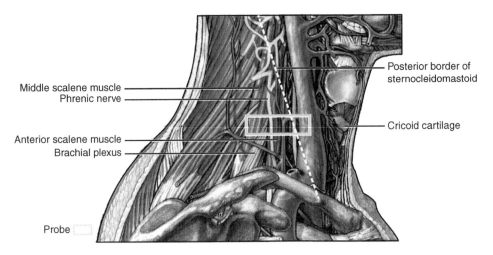

Middle scalene muscle
Phrenic nerve
Anterior scalene muscle
Brachial plexus
Posterior border of sternocleidomastoid
Cricoid cartilage
Probe

Fig 3.1 **Lateral neck (sternocleidomastoid muscle removed)**

Probe placement for interscalene brachial plexus block

Position the patient supine with the head turned towards the contralateral side. Use a linear probe at the level of the cricoid cartilage in a coronal plane.

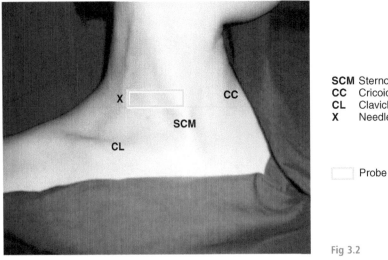

SCM Sternocleidomastoid
CC Cricoid cartilage
CL Clavicle
X Needle entry point

Probe

Fig 3.2

Scan of interscalene brachial plexus

The nerve roots appear as hypoechoic dark round structures between the scalene muscles. The internal jugular vein and carotid artery are seen deep to these structures.

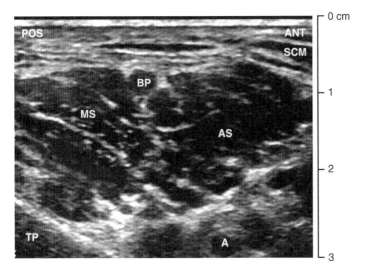

SCM	Sternocleidomastoid
MS	Middle scalene muscle
AS	Anterior scalene
BP	Brachial plexus
A	Vertebral artery
TP	Transverse process

Fig 3.3

Diagram of scan

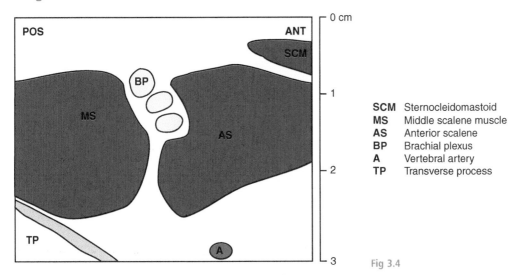

SCM	Sternocleidomastoid
MS	Middle scalene muscle
AS	Anterior scalene
BP	Brachial plexus
A	Vertebral artery
TP	Transverse process

Fig 3.4

Tips and complications Use an in-plane technique for injections because this reduces the risk of unintentional deep injections. An out-of-plane technique may be required for catheter insertion. If the nerve roots in the interscalene space are difficult to identify, track the brachial plexus nerves upwards from their supraclavicular position. The phrenic nerve lies on the anterior surface of the anterior scalene muscle and is commonly anaesthetized during an interscalene block. Needling from the posterior aspect of the probe when in plane reduces this risk. Injections which are too deep may result in intravascular injection or neuraxial anaesthesia.

Anatomy of the infraclavicular brachial plexus

The brachial plexus enters the infraclavicular region from the posterior triangle of the neck by passing across the first rib under cover of the clavicle. In the infraclavicular region, the brachial plexus (C5–T1) is in the form of the lateral, medial and posterior cords. These lie in close proximity to the axillary artery and vein, deep to the pectoralis major and minor muscles.

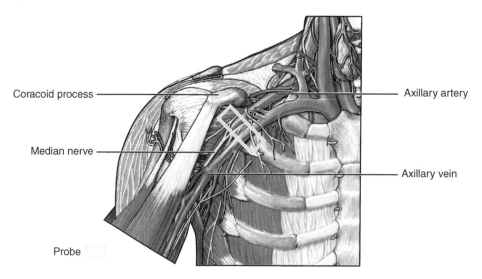

Coracoid process

Median nerve

Probe

Axillary artery

Axillary vein

Fig 4.1

Probe placement for infraclavicular brachial plexus block

Position the patient supine with the arm to be blocked at the patient's side. A linear probe can be used in smaller patients, while a curvilinear probe may be needed in larger patients. Apply the probe 4–6 cm caudal to the coracoid process, roughly parallel to the clavicle, so that the plane of the ultrasound beam cuts across the brachial plexus cords and axillary vessels.

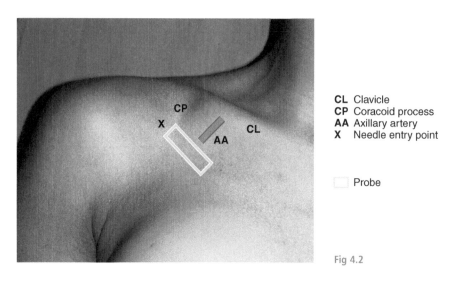

CL Clavicle
CP Coracoid process
AA Axillary artery
X Needle entry point

Probe

Fig 4.2

18

Scan of infraclavicular brachial plexus

The main landmarks in this scan are the axillary vessels and the pectoralis major and minor muscles. The cords of the brachial plexus are distributed around the axillary artery and may not be easily identifiable because of their depth.

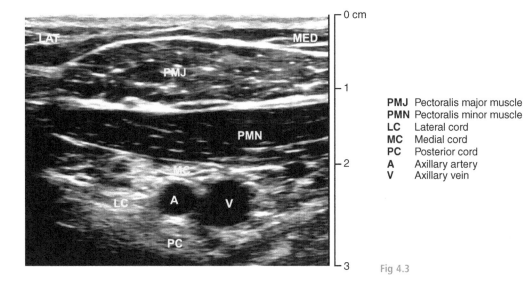

Fig 4.3

PMJ Pectoralis major muscle
PMN Pectoralis minor muscle
LC   Lateral cord
MC   Medial cord
PC   Posterior cord
A   Axillary artery
V   Axillary vein

Diagram of scan

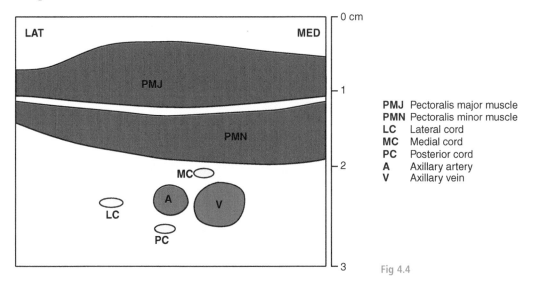

Fig 4.4

PMJ Pectoralis major muscle
PMN Pectoralis minor muscle
LC   Lateral cord
MC   Medial cord
PC   Posterior cord
A   Axillary artery
V   Axillary vein

Tips and complications Abduction of the arm to 90 degrees will bring the three cords closer together and enhance nerve visualization. An in-plane approach is recommended from the cephalad end of the probe along its long axis. Obtaining local anaesthetic spread to the posterior cord may be difficult. Puncture of the axillary vessels and the chest wall are the main hazards.

Anatomy of the axillary brachial plexus

The terminal branches of the brachial plexus are the median (C6–T1), ulnar (C7–T1) and radial (C5–T1) nerves. These are located superficially in the axilla and are adjacent to the axillary artery and vein(s). This neurovascular bundle lies in a space between two muscle masses. The biceps, together with coracobrachialis, lies anteriorly, while the triceps lies posteriorly. The musculocutaneous nerve (C5–C7) leaves the lateral cord high in the axilla to lie in the plane between biceps and coracobrachialis.

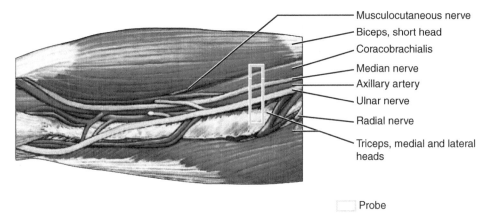

- Musculocutaneous nerve
- Biceps, short head
- Coracobrachialis
- Median nerve
- Axillary artery
- Ulnar nerve
- Radial nerve
- Triceps, medial and lateral heads

☐ Probe

Fig 5.1

Probe placement for axillary brachial plexus block

Position the patient supine with the arm abducted to 90 degrees, externally rotated, and the elbow flexed. Identify the axillary artery lying between the biceps (with coracobrachialis) and triceps muscle. Position a linear probe transversely across the axillary arterial pulse.

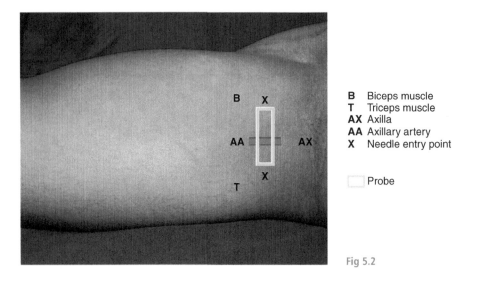

B Biceps muscle
T Triceps muscle
AX Axilla
AA Axillary artery
X Needle entry point

☐ Probe

Fig 5.2

Scan of axillary brachial plexus

The axillary artery is the most prominent landmark in the scan. Nerve echogenicity is heterogeneous and they have a honeycomb appearance. Axillary veins are distinguished from the artery by their compressibility.

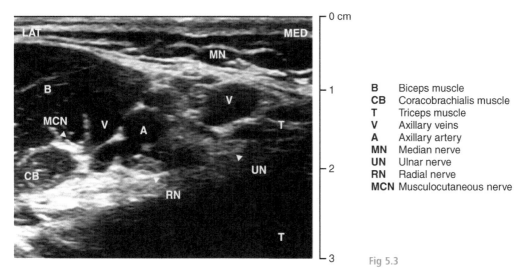

B   Biceps muscle
CB   Coracobrachialis muscle
T   Triceps muscle
V   Axillary veins
A   Axillary artery
MN   Median nerve
UN   Ulnar nerve
RN   Radial nerve
MCN Musculocutaneous nerve

Fig 5.3

Diagram of scan

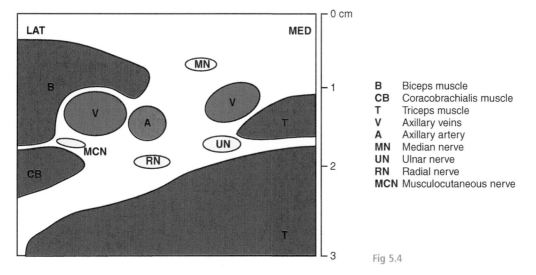

B   Biceps muscle
CB   Coracobrachialis muscle
T   Triceps muscle
V   Axillary veins
A   Axillary artery
MN   Median nerve
UN   Ulnar nerve
RN   Radial nerve
MCN Musculocutaneous nerve

Fig 5.4

Tips and complications The axillary brachial plexus block is best performed using an in-line technique, usually approaching from the lateral side of the probe for the median and musculocutaneous nerves, while a medial approach is used for the ulnar and radial nerves. The radial nerve is the most difficult to locate, being deep to the axillary artery and lying on the surface of the triceps fascia. Direct the needle to the space between biceps and coracobrachialis to block the musculocutaneous nerve. Complications include injection into the axillary vessels.

Anatomy of the radial nerve in the upper arm

The radial nerve (C5–T1) is the largest terminal branch of the posterior cord. It enters the upper arm lying between the lateral and medial heads of triceps and descends in the radial groove of the humerus. As it approaches the elbow it perforates the lateral intermuscular septum and enters the cubital fossa, where it divides into deep and superficial branches. The deep branch is a motor nerve, perforating the interosseous membrane as the posterior interosseous nerve of the forearm, and supplies the muscles in the posterior compartment. The superficial branch is sensory and passes into the forearm to supply skin over the dorsolateral aspect of the hand and wrist.

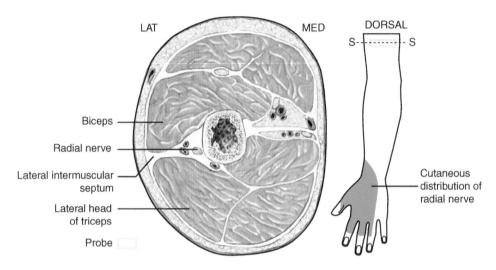

Fig 6.1 **Upper arm (cross-section at SS)**

Probe placement for radial nerve block in upper arm

Place a linear probe transversely across the lateral aspect of the upper arm at the junction of the lower and middle thirds. Track the radial nerve as it passes distally in the radial groove between the lateral and medial heads of triceps.

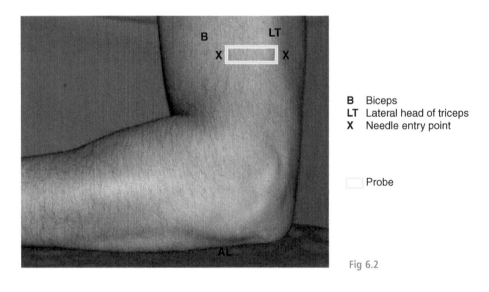

B Biceps
LT Lateral head of triceps
X Needle entry point

Probe

Fig 6.2

Scan of radial nerve in upper arm

The radial nerve is readily identified when applying a linear probe to the lateral aspect of the upper arm, as it lies in the radial groove of the humerus. Tracking the nerve distally, it can be seen to 'lift' away from the humerus as the lateral epicondyle and the elbow are approached.

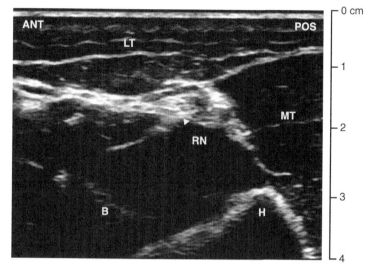

B   Brachialis
LT Lateral head of triceps
MT Medial head of triceps
RN Radial nerve
H   Humerus

Fig 6.3

Diagram of scan

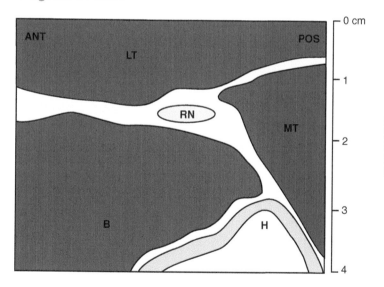

B   Brachialis
LT Lateral head of triceps
MT Medial head of triceps
RN Radial nerve
H   Humerus

Fig 6.4

Tips and complications Use an in-plane technique for single-shot blocks, but for catheter insertion out of plane is easiest. Nerve stimulation can be used to confirm nerve identity, as the nerve at this level contains a motor component producing dorsiflexion of the wrist.

23

Anatomy of the medial cutaneous nerve of the forearm

The medial cutaneous nerve of the forearm (C8, T1) is a purely sensory nerve, and is the smallest branch of the brachial plexus. It originates from the medial cord in the infraclavicular region. This nerve passes distally with the brachial vessels and the median and ulnar nerves, becoming subcutaneous in the mid upper arm. It joins a branch from the ulnar nerve and passes across the cubital fossa in close relation to the median cubital vein, to supply an area of skin over the medial forearm, which extends from the elbow to the wrist. Figure 7.1 illustrates the subcutaneous structures over the cubital fossa area.

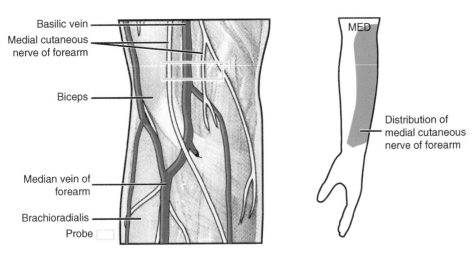

Fig 7.1

Probe placement for block of medial cutaneous nerve of forearm

Use a linear probe placed across the basilic vein above the elbow joint and over the medial aspect of the upper arm.

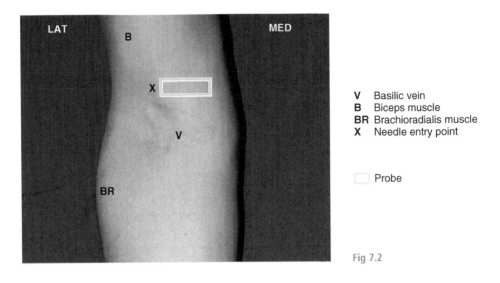

V   Basilic vein
B   Biceps muscle
BR Brachioradialis muscle
X   Needle entry point

☐ Probe

Fig 7.2

Scan of medial cutaneous nerve of forearm

The basilic vein is used as a vascular landmark, and this can be identified as a superficial vein over the medial aspect of the upper arm, which overlies the biceps and brachialis muscles. The lateral cutaneous nerve of the forearm can usually be found between the basilic vein and biceps/brachialis.

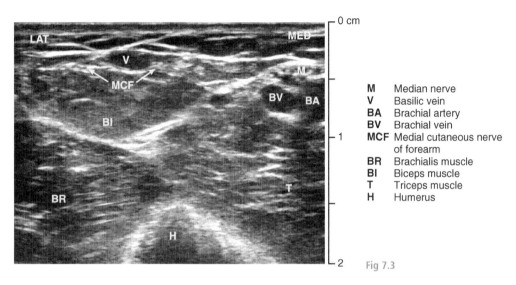

M   Median nerve
V   Basilic vein
BA   Brachial artery
BV   Brachial vein
MCF Medial cutaneous nerve
     of forearm
BR   Brachialis muscle
BI   Biceps muscle
T   Triceps muscle
H   Humerus

Fig 7.3

Diagram of scan

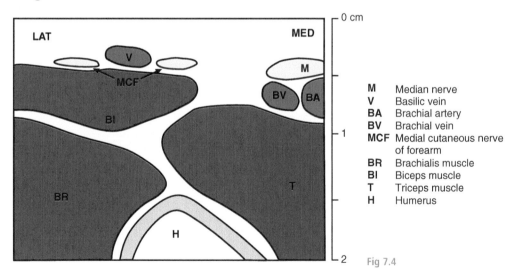

M   Median nerve
V   Basilic vein
BA   Brachial artery
BV   Brachial vein
MCF Medial cutaneous nerve
     of forearm
BR   Brachialis muscle
BI   Biceps muscle
T   Triceps muscle
H   Humerus

Fig 7.4

Tips and complications Insert the needle in plane to avoid puncture of the basilic vein. Use a nerve stimulator to confirm proximity of the needle tip for radiofrequency lesioning.

Anatomy of the lateral cutaneous nerve of the forearm

The lateral cutaneous nerve of the forearm (C5, C6) is the terminal continuation of the musculocutaneous nerve. The musculocutaneous nerve originates from the lateral cord of the brachial plexus in the infraclavicular region. It passes distally in the space between coracobrachialis and biceps, and emerges subcutaneously just proximal to the elbow joint, lateral to brachialis and the median vein. It supplies an area of skin over the brachioradialis muscle in the lateral forearm, which extends from the cubital fossa to the wrist.

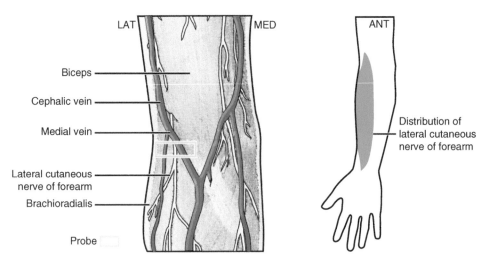

Fig 8.1

Probe placement for block of lateral cutaneous nerve of forearm

Use a linear probe placed over the median vein in the cubital fossa, overlying the upper part of the brachioradialis muscle.

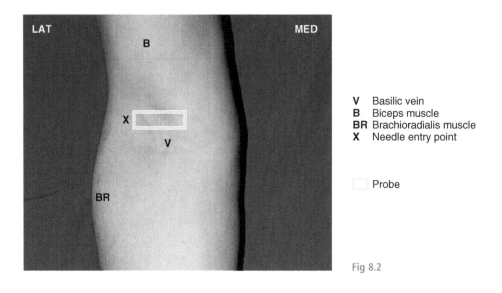

V   Basilic vein
B   Biceps muscle
BR   Brachioradialis muscle
X   Needle entry point

    Probe

Fig 8.2

Scan of lateral cutaneous nerve of forearm

The median vein is used as a vascular landmark, and this can often be identified in the cubital fossa, over the anterior aspect of the elbow joint. Lateral to this vein is the brachioradialis muscle. The lateral cutaneous nerve of the forearm can usually be found between the median vein and brachioradialis.

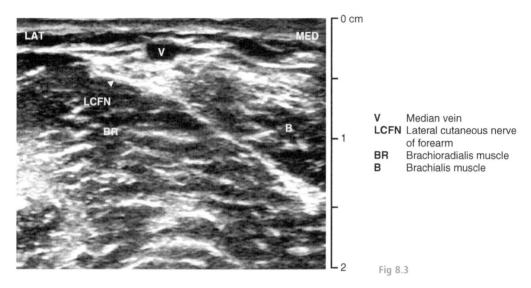

V	Median vein
LCFN	Lateral cutaneous nerve of forearm
BR	Brachioradialis muscle
B	Brachialis muscle

Fig 8.3

Diagram of scan

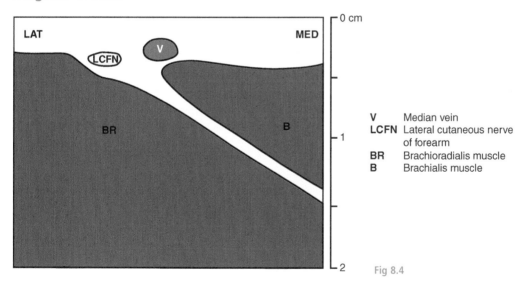

V	Median vein
LCFN	Lateral cutaneous nerve of forearm
BR	Brachioradialis muscle
B	Brachialis muscle

Fig 8.4

Tips and complications Insert the needle in plane to avoid puncture of the median vein. Use a nerve stimulator to confirm proximity of the needle tip for radiofrequency lesioning.

Anatomy of the median nerve in the cubital fossa

The median nerve (C5–T1) is derived from both the lateral and medial cords. It descends lateral to the brachial artery in the upper arm and crosses over to lie medial to the artery as it approaches the elbow joint. In the cubital fossa the median nerve remains immediately medial to the brachial artery and anterior to the brachialis muscle. It exits from the cubital fossa deep to the bicipital aponeurosis and pronator teres muscle, and enters the forearm. The median nerve provides the motor supply to the flexor muscles of the forearm except for flexor carpi ulnaris and the medial half of flexor digitorum profundus. It also supplies the intrinsic muscles of the thumb and sensation to the lateral three and a half digits.

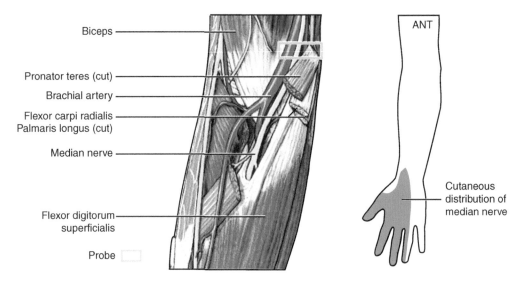

Fig 9.1

Probe placement for median nerve block in cubital fossa

Identify the cubital fossa. The superior border is a line joining the medial and lateral epicondyles, the medial border is pronator teres and the lateral border is brachioradialis. Find the brachial artery pulse in the medial side of the fossa, and place the probe transversely over the pulse.

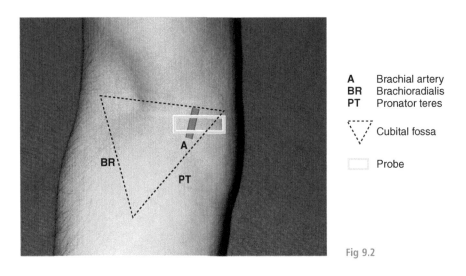

A   Brachial artery
BR Brachioradialis
PT Pronator teres

Cubital fossa

Probe

Fig 9.2

Scan of median nerve in cubital fossa

In this scan the brachial artery is the main landmark. Immediately medial to this lies the median nerve. Track the nerve distally as it exits the cubital fossa deep to pronator teres, to enter the space between flexor digitorum superficialis and flexor digitorum profundus in the forearm.

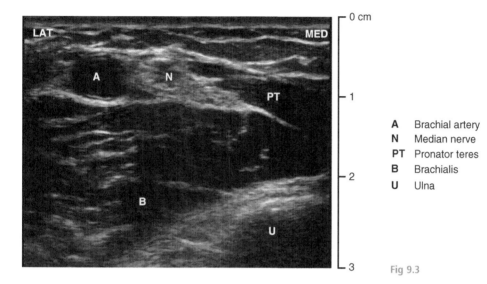

A	Brachial artery
N	Median nerve
PT	Pronator teres
B	Brachialis
U	Ulna

Fig 9.3

Diagram of scan

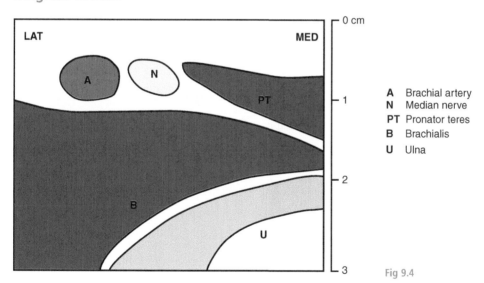

A	Brachial artery
N	Median nerve
PT	Pronator teres
B	Brachialis
U	Ulna

Fig 9.4

Tips and complications Insert the needle from the medial aspect of the probe to reduce chances of perforating the brachial artery.

Anatomy of the median nerve in the forearm

The median nerve (C5–T1) is derived from the lateral and medial cords of the brachial plexus. It enters the forearm deep to the pronator teres and flexor digitorum superficialis muscles. In the forearm its course lies in the plane between flexor digitorum superficialis and flexor digitorum profundus. The median nerve is a mixed nerve, providing the motor supply to the flexors of the anterior forearm compartment (except for flexor carpi ulnaris and the medial half of flexor digitorum superficialis). The terminal branches of the median nerve pass into the hand to supply some of the muscles of the hand and the skin of the lateral palm and lateral (radial) three and a half digits.

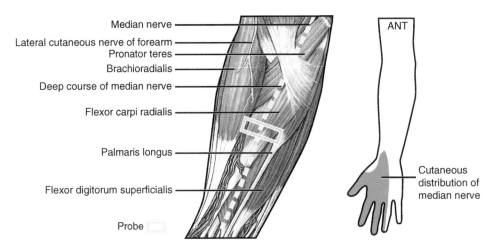

Median nerve
Lateral cutaneous nerve of forearm
Pronator teres
Brachioradialis
Deep course of median nerve
Flexor carpi radialis
Palmaris longus
Flexor digitorum superficialis
Probe

ANT

Cutaneous distribution of median nerve

Fig 10.1

Probe placement for median nerve block in forearm

Place a linear probe transversely across mid forearm with its centre over flexor carpi radialis and palmaris longus muscles. Identify these superficial flexors by asking the patient to flex the wrist.

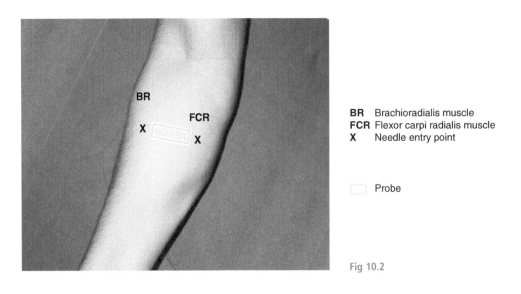

BR
FCR
X   X

BR Brachioradialis muscle
FCR Flexor carpi radialis muscle
X Needle entry point

Probe

Fig 10.2

Scan of median nerve in forearm

There are no convenient vascular or bony landmarks to identify the median nerve in the mid forearm, but the nerve is usually readily visible as a hyperechoic target in the surrounding muscles. Track the median nerve either proximally from the wrist or distally from the cubital fossa. At this level in the forearm the superficial branch of the radial nerve with the radial artery can often be seen lateral to the median nerve.

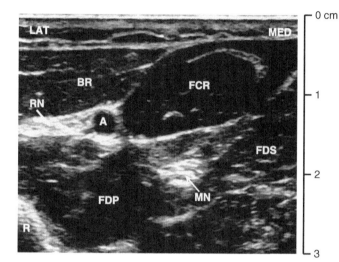

FCR	Flexor carpi radialis
BR	Brachioradialis
FDP	Flexor digitorum profundus
FDS	Flexor digitorum superficialis
A	Radial artery
RN	Radial nerve
MN	Median nerve
R	Radius

Fig 10.3

Diagram of scan

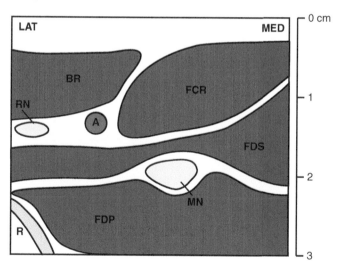

FCR	Flexor carpi radialis
BR	Brachioradialis
FDP	Flexor digitorum profundus
FDS	Flexor digitorum superficialis
A	Radial artery
RN	Radial nerve
MN	Median nerve
R	Radius

Fig 10.4

Tips and complications At this level the median nerve is not close to an artery, so the risk of unwanted vascular puncture is reduced. This level of the forearm is suitable for catheter insertion for infusion blockade. Confirm identity of the nerve by tracking it from the wrist or using a nerve stimulator.

Anatomy of the ulnar nerve in the forearm

The ulnar nerve is the terminal branch of the medial cord, formed from C8 and T1 (and often fibres from C7). It enters the forearm from the ulnar groove posterior to the medial epicondyle, by passing between the two heads of flexor carpi ulnaris. In the forearm the ulnar nerve lies on the surface of flexor digitorum profundus, deep to the flexor carpi ulnaris and flexor digitorum superficialis muscles. The ulnar nerve is a mixed nerve supplying flexor carpi ulnaris and the medial half of flexor digitorum superficialis in the forearm. It then passes distally to supply small muscles of the hand and skin over the medial palm and medial one and a half fingers.

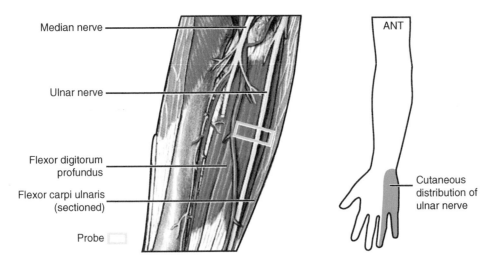

Median nerve

Ulnar nerve

Flexor digitorum profundus

Flexor carpi ulnaris (sectioned)

Probe

ANT

Cutaneous distribution of ulnar nerve

Fig 11.1

Probe placement for ulnar nerve block in forearm

Abduct the patient's arm to 90 degrees and flex it at the elbow. This manoeuvre causes the arm to rotate externally, improving access to the medial aspect of the forearm. Identify flexor carpi ulnaris by asking the patient to flex the wrist towards the ulnar side. Place a linear probe transversely across flexor carpi ulnaris.

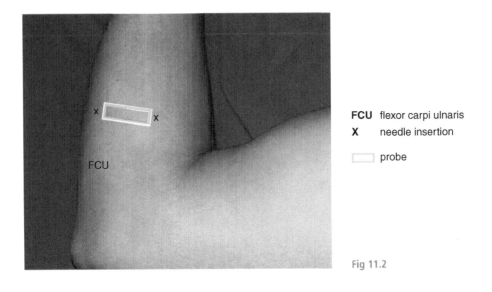

FCU

FCU flexor carpi ulnaris

X needle insertion

▭ probe

Fig 11.2

Scan of ulnar nerve in forearm

The ulnar artery is a convenient vascular landmark. The ulnar nerve is usually medial to the artery.

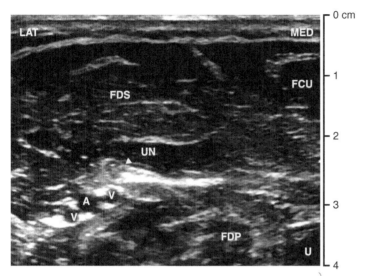

FDS Flexor digitorum superficialis
FCU Flexor carpi ulnaris
FDP Flexor digitorum profundus
UN   Ulnar nerve
A   Ulnar artery
V   Veins accompanying artery
U   Ulna

Fig 11.3

Diagram of scan

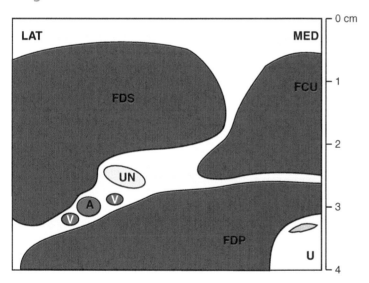

FDS Flexor digitorum superficialis
FCU Flexor carpi ulnaris
FDP Flexor digitorum profundus
UN   Ulnar nerve
A   Ulnar artery
V   Veins accompanying artery
U   Ulna

Fig 11.4

Tips and complications If the ulnar nerve is not easily identified, locate it at the wrist where it lies between the ulnar artery and the flexor carpi ulnaris tendon. Track it proximally until it begins to diverge from the ulnar artery, where it can be blocked with reduced risk of puncturing the ulnar vessels. Use an in-plane technique for single-shot blocks, but for catheter insertion out of plane is easiest. Nerve stimulation can be used to confirm nerve identity.

Anatomy of the superficial radial nerve in the forearm

The radial nerve (C5–T1) is the larger terminal branch of the posterior cord, and enters the cubital fossa from between brachialis and brachioradialis, lying anterior to the lateral epicondyle. In the cubital fossa the radial nerve divides into deep and superficial branches. The deep branch (posterior interosseous nerve) perforates the interosseous septum to supply the muscles in the posterior compartment of the forearm. The superficial branch is sensory, entering the forearm to lie under the brachioradialis muscle, and crosses over supinator, pronator teres and flexor digitorum superficialis as it passes distally from elbow to wrist.

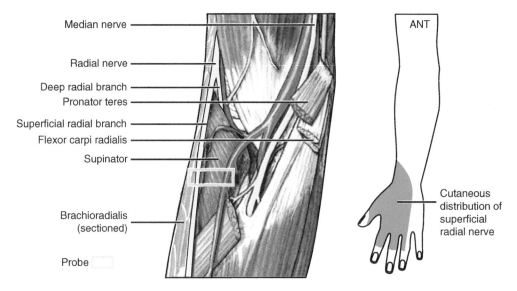

Fig 12.1

Probe placement for superficial radial nerve block in forearm

Place a linear probe transversely across the lateral aspect of the forearm. Position the probe over the brachioradialis muscle, which can be located by asking the awake patient to flex the elbow against resistance.

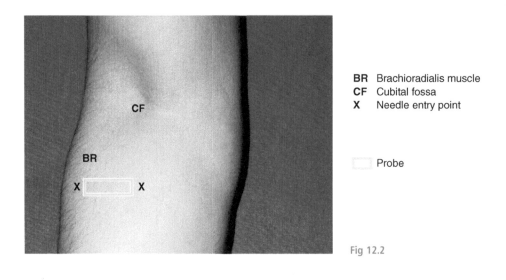

BR Brachioradialis muscle
CF Cubital fossa
X Needle entry point

Probe

Fig 12.2

Scan of superficial radial nerve in forearm

The radial artery is a convenient vascular landmark in this scan. The radial nerve lies lateral to the radial artery. Its identity can be confirmed by tracking the nerve to the radial aspect of the wrist.

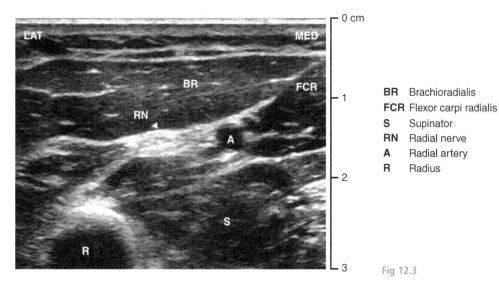

BR	Brachioradialis
FCR	Flexor carpi radialis
S	Supinator
RN	Radial nerve
A	Radial artery
R	Radius

Fig 12.3

Diagram of scan

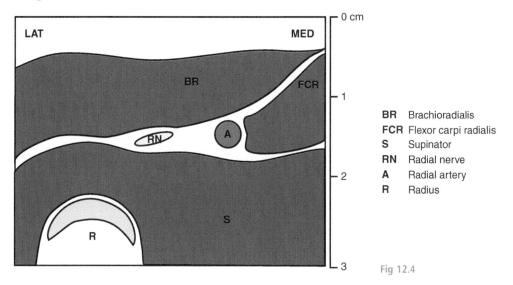

BR	Brachioradialis
FCR	Flexor carpi radialis
S	Supinator
RN	Radial nerve
A	Radial artery
R	Radius

Fig 12.4

Tips and complications This level of the forearm is optimal for catheter insertion if prolonged regional blockade in the hand is required. Nerve stimulation can be used to confirm nerve identity. Insert the needle out of plane for catheter placement.

35

Anatomy of the median nerve at the wrist

The median nerve enters the wrist from the space between the flexor digitorum superficialis and flexor digitorum profundus muscles. It becomes superficial in the midline of the wrist, lying between the flexor carpi radialis tendon laterally (radial side) and the palmaris longus tendon medially (ulnar side), before entering the palm of the hand in a sheath deep to the flexor retinaculum. Proximal to the wrist creases it gives off a palmar cutaneous branch which passes over the flexor retinaculum to supply sensation to the lateral palm. The median nerve is a mixed nerve, supplying the muscles of the thenar eminence, the lateral two lumbricals, and sensation to the lateral three and a half fingers. Constriction or compression in its sheath gives rise to carpal tunnel syndrome.

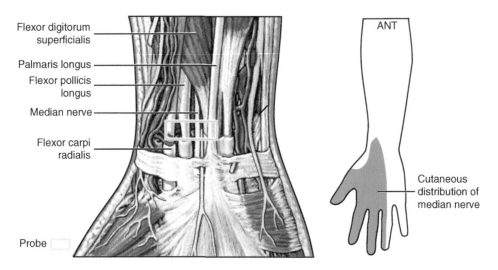

Flexor digitorum superficialis

Palmaris longus

Flexor pollicis longus

Median nerve

Flexor carpi radialis

Probe

ANT

Cutaneous distribution of median nerve

Fig 13.1

Probe placement for median nerve block at wrist

A small linear or hockey-stick probe is placed transversely over the space between the palmaris longus and flexor carpi radialis tendons at the proximal wrist crease. Identify these tendons by asking the patient to flex the wrist.

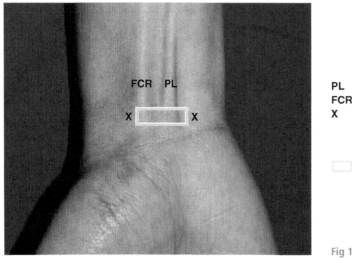

FCR   PL

X   X

PL   Palmaris longus tendon
FCR Flexor carpi radialis tendon
X   Needle entry point

Probe

Fig 13.2

Scan of median nerve at wrist

It may be difficult to distinguish the median nerve from adjacent tendons, but when traced proximally the tendons will turn to muscle belly, while the median nerve remains unchanged and descends deeper to lie between the flexor digitorum superficialis and flexor digitorum profundus muscles.

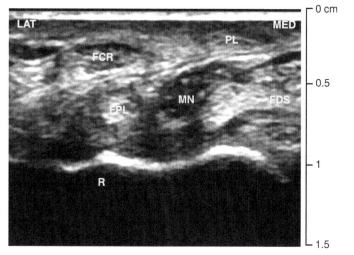

PL   Palmaris longus tendon
FCR Flexor carpi radialis tendon
FPL Flexor pollicis longus tendon
FDS Flexor digitorum superficialis
      tendons
MN Median nerve
R   Radius

Fig 13.3

Diagram of scan

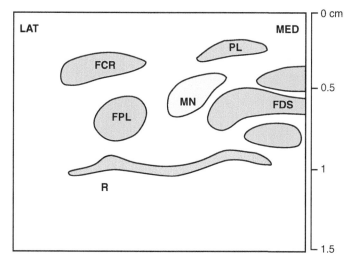

PL   Palmaris longus tendon
FCR Flexor carpi radialis tendon
FPL Flexor pollicis longus tendon
FDS Flexor digitorum superficialis
       tendons
MN   Median nerve
R   Radius

Fig 13.4

Tips and complications Correct identification of the nerve, differentiating it from adjacent tendons, can be difficult when scanning. Identify the flexor carpi radialis and palmaris longus tendons by asking the patient to flex the wrist. Similarly the flexor digitorum superficialis tendons will move with flexion of the fingers at the metacarpophalangeal joints.

Anatomy of the ulnar nerve at the wrist

The ulnar nerve (C8, T1 and occasionally C7) lies between the flexor digitorum profundus, flexor digitorum superficialis and flexor carpi ulnaris muscles in the forearm. It enters the wrist from this space, and is a mixed nerve passing into the hand superficial to the flexor retinaculum, to supply the small muscles of the hand (except for the thenar eminence and the lateral two lumbricals). It supplies sensation to the lateral palm and the lateral one and a half fingers. At the wrist the ulnar nerve usually lies between the ulnar artery and the flexor carpi ulnaris tendon.

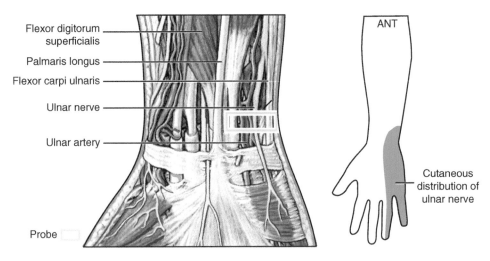

Flexor digitorum superficialis
Palmaris longus
Flexor carpi ulnaris
Ulnar nerve
Ulnar artery
Probe

ANT
Cutaneous distribution of ulnar nerve

Fig 14.1

Probe placement for ulnar nerve block at wrist

At the proximal wrist crease, locate the ulnar arterial pulse and identify the flexor carpi ulnaris tendon by asking the patient to flex the wrist to the ulnar side. Place a small linear or hockey-stick probe across the ulnar artery and flexor carpi ulnaris tendon.

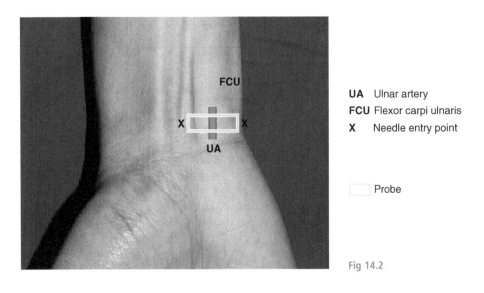

FCU
X   X
UA

UA Ulnar artery
FCU Flexor carpi ulnaris
X   Needle entry point

Probe

Fig 14.2

Scan of ulnar nerve at wrist

The ulnar artery is a convenient vascular landmark in the scan. The ulnar nerve lies immediately medial to the artery and lateral or deep to the tendon of flexor carpi ulnaris.

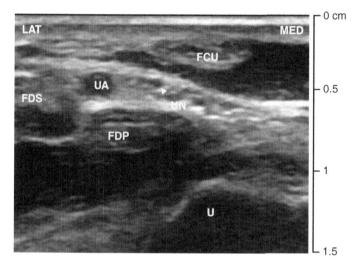

FCU	Flexor carpi ulnaris tendon
FDS	Flexor digitorum superficialis
FDP	Flexor digitorum profundus
UN	Ulnar nerve
UA	Ulnar artery
U	Ulna

Fig 14.3

Diagram of scan

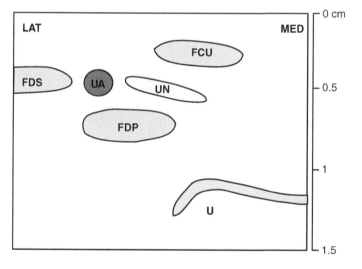

FCU	Flexor carpi ulnaris tendon
FDS	Flexor digitorum superficialis
FDP	Flexor digitorum profundus
UN	Ulnar nerve
UA	Ulnar artery
U	Ulna

Fig 14.4

Tips and complications The nerve is often difficult to differentiate from the tendons nearby in the wrist. Identify the tendons by their movement when the patient is asked to flex the wrist to the medial side. Also ask the patient to flex the fingers at the metacarpophalangeal joint to identify the tendons of flexor digitorum superficialis. Track the ulnar nerve and ulnar artery proximally into the forearm, where they will stay next to each other in the space between flexor carpi ulnaris and flexor digitorum profundus. In the proximal third of the forearm the artery and nerve separate, making it easier to block the ulnar nerve without risk of arterial puncture.

Anatomy of the femoral nerve

The femoral nerve (L2,3,4) emerges from under the inguinal ligament to lie lateral to the femoral artery. It is a mixed motor and sensory nerve. The main motor supply is to the quadriceps femoris, which has a primary action of extending the knee joint. It also supplies pectineus, iliacus and sartorius. The sensory component covers the anterior and distal medial thigh. The femoral nerve lies within the iliopsoas compartment and not within the femoral sheath.

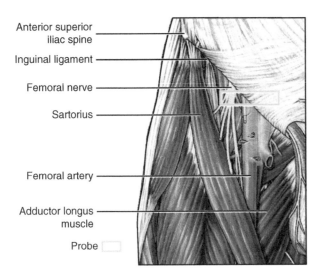
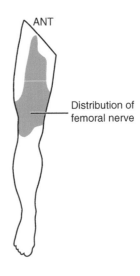

Anterior superior iliac spine

Inguinal ligament

Femoral nerve

Sartorius

Femoral artery

Adductor longus muscle

Probe

ANT

Distribution of femoral nerve

Fig 15.1

Probe placement for femoral nerve block

Use the borders of the femoral triangle (superior = inguinal ligament, lateral = sartorius muscle, medial = adductor longus) and position the probe across the femoral artery.

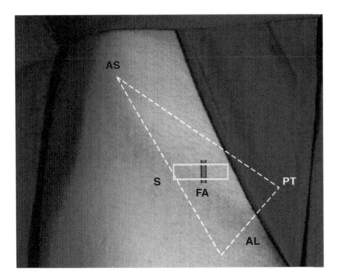

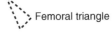

AS Anterior superior iliac spine
PT Pubic tubercle
FA Femoral artery
S Sartorius muscle
AL Adductor longus muscle
X Needle entry point

Probe

Femoral triangle

Fig 15.2

Scan of femoral nerve

Use the femoral artery and vein as landmarks. Identify the femoral vein by compression and the iliopectineal fascia. The femoral nerve lies lateral to the artery immediately beneath the iliopectineal fascia.

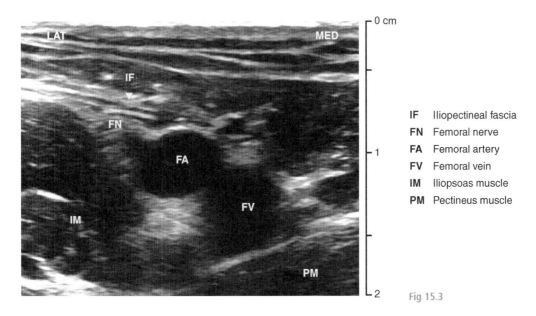

IF   Iliopectineal fascia
FN   Femoral nerve
FA   Femoral artery
FV   Femoral vein
IM   Iliopsoas muscle
PM   Pectineus muscle

Fig 15.3

Diagram of scan

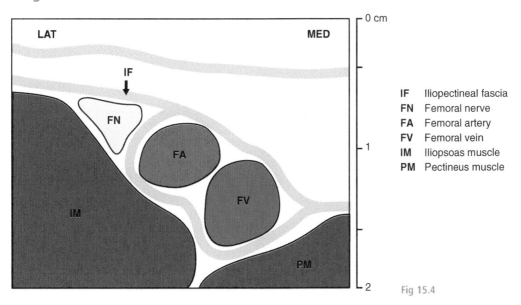

IF   Iliopectineal fascia
FN   Femoral nerve
FA   Femoral artery
FV   Femoral vein
IM   Iliopsoas muscle
PM   Pectineus muscle

Fig 15.4

Tips and complications Needle insertion is made in plane and lateral to the probe to avoid the femoral vessels. The femoral nerve lies within the iliopsoas muscle compartment and the needle must therefore pass through two fascial layers, the fascia lata and the iliopectineal fascia (two 'pops') in order to reach the nerve. Visualize the local anaesthetic spread directly, because if the iliopectineal fascia is not pierced the local anaesthetic can spread away from the nerve resulting in a poor block. The nerve may be better visualized once a small amount of local anaesthetic has been deposited around it. The posterior branch of the femoral nerve may be found above iliopsoas and more lateral to the femoral artery than expected. This is a relatively well tolerated superficial nerve block, the main complications of which are intravascular and intraneural injection of local anaesthetic.

Anatomy of the lateral cutaneous nerve of the thigh

The lateral cutaneous nerve of the thigh (LCNT) is derived from spinal roots L2 and L3 of the lumbar plexus. It is a sensory nerve supplying sensation to skin over the anterolateral aspects of the thigh. The nerve passes through the inguinal ligament immediately medial to the anterior superior iliac spine (ASIS), coming to lie on the surface of sartorius. It passes through a hiatus in the attachment of the inguinal ligament to the ASIS.

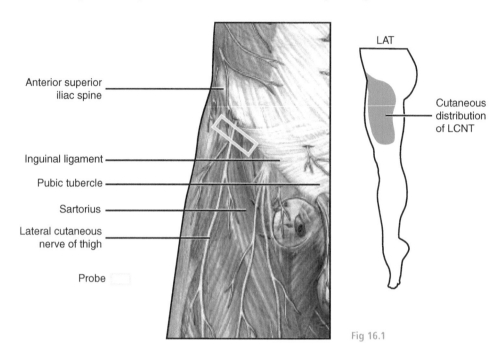

Fig 16.1

Probe placement for block of lateral cutaneous nerve of thigh

Identify the anterior superior iliac spine (ASIS), the pubic tubercle and the inguinal ligament, which passes from the ASIS to attach to the pubic tubercle. Place a linear probe caudal to the ASIS oriented parallel to the inguinal ligament, so that it lies over the sartorius muscle.

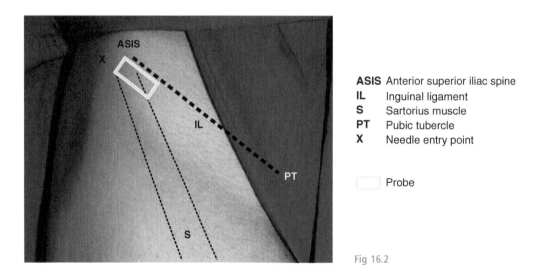

ASIS Anterior superior iliac spine
IL Inguinal ligament
S Sartorius muscle
PT Pubic tubercle
X Needle entry point

☐ Probe

Fig 16.2

Scan of lateral cutaneous nerve of thigh

The subcutaneous fascia of the sartorius muscle can be identified easily on the scan. The LCNT can be seen just deep to the sartorius fascia on the surface of the muscle.

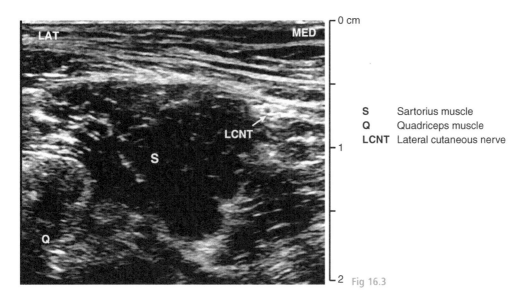

S	Sartorius muscle
Q	Quadriceps muscle
LCNT	Lateral cutaneous nerve

Fig 16.3

Diagram of scan

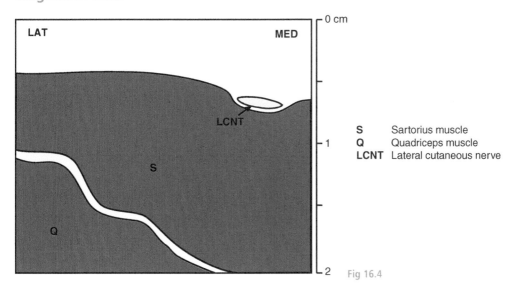

S	Sartorius muscle
Q	Quadriceps muscle
LCNT	Lateral cutaneous nerve

Fig 16.4

Tips and complications The LCNT is a peripheral nerve which is not easily seen. A simple block can be obtained by passing the needle through the sartorius fascia and injecting into the sartorius compartment. A stimulator may be useful to confirm identity of the LCNT for radiofrequency lesioning. Puncture of the femoral vessels can be avoided by scanning the probe medially first to identify these vessels, and ensuring that the probe is lateral to the femoral triangle.

43

Anatomy of the obturator nerve

The obturator nerve (L2,3,4) is a mixed motor and sensory nerve. The motor supply is to the three adductor muscles of the thigh – adductor longus (AL), adductor brevis (AB), adductor magnus (AM) – and gracilis. The sensory supply covers an area over the medial thigh extending to the knee, and also has an articular branch to the knee joint capsule. The obturator nerve emerges from the pelvis via the obturator foramen, splitting into anterior and posterior divisions before entering the thigh. In the thigh these divisions are separated by AB. The anterior division lies between AL and AB, while the posterior division lies between AB and AM.

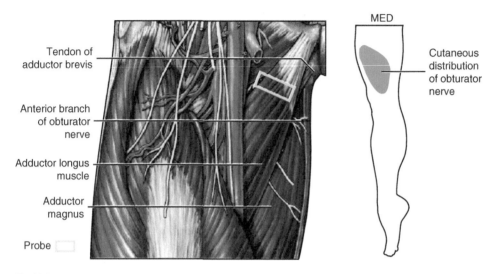

Fig 17.1

Probe placement for obturator nerve block

Identify the adductor longus, which forms the medial border of the femoral triangle, and place a linear probe over the body of the muscle.

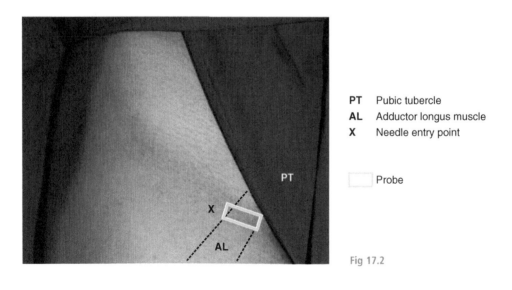

PT   Pubic tubercle
AL   Adductor longus muscle
X   Needle entry point

☐   Probe

Fig 17.2

Scan of obturator nerve

Identify the three adductor muscle layers in the scan: adductor longus (the most superficial), adductor brevis and adductor magnus (the deepest layer). The fascial planes between these muscles are the potential spaces to be injected with local anaesthetic in order to block the anterior and posterior divisions of the obturator nerve.

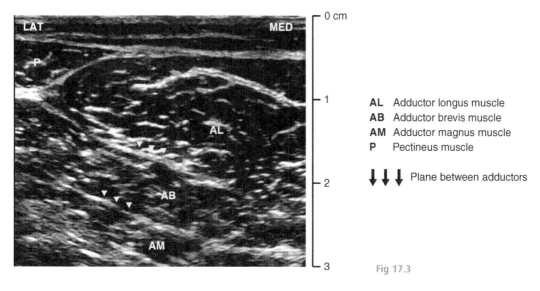

AL   Adductor longus muscle
AB   Adductor brevis muscle
AM   Adductor magnus muscle
P   Pectineus muscle

↓ ↓ ↓   Plane between adductors

Fig 17.3

Diagram of scan

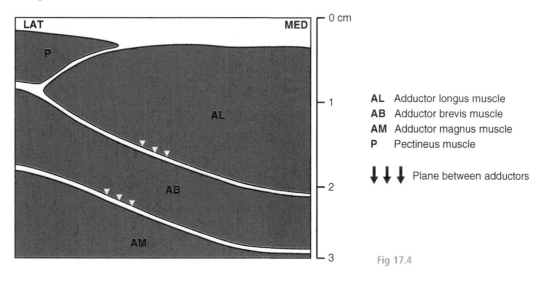

AL   Adductor longus muscle
AB   Adductor brevis muscle
AM   Adductor magnus muscle
P   Pectineus muscle

↓ ↓ ↓   Plane between adductors

Fig 17.4

Tips and complications Puncture of the femoral vessels is a possible complication.

Anatomy of the sciatic nerve in the gluteal region

The sciatic nerve is the largest nerve in the body and originates from the anterior rami of L4,5, S1,2,3. It provides the motor supply to the flexors of the knee in the thigh, and all of the muscles of the lower leg and foot, as well as some articular branches to the hip joint. The cutaneous distribution of the sciatic nerve covers the lower leg and foot, apart from the medial aspect, which is the territory of the saphenous nerve (L2,3,4). It enters the gluteal region via the greater sciatic notch, passing below the piriformis muscle to lie between the ischial tuberosity and the greater trochanter.

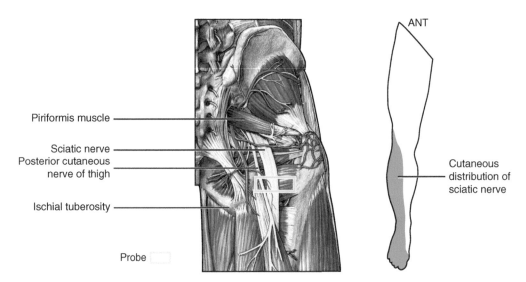

Piriformis muscle

Sciatic nerve
Posterior cutaneous
nerve of thigh

Ischial tuberosity

Probe

ANT

Cutaneous
distribution of
sciatic nerve

Fig 18.1

Probe placement for sciatic nerve block at gluteal fold

Identify the greater trochanter and the ischial tuberosity. An ultrasound probe is then placed halfway between these landmarks.

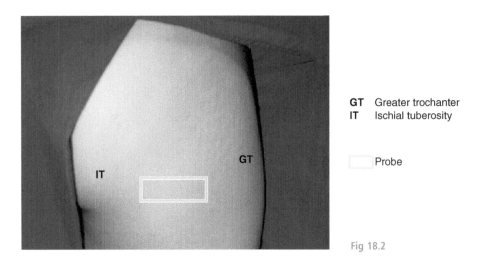

GT Greater trochanter
IT   Ischial tuberosity

Probe

GT

IT

Fig 18.2

Scan of sciatic nerve at gluteal fold

At this level the sciatic nerve lies between gluteus maximus and quadratus femoris in a potential space, the subgluteal space. It is accompanied on the medial side by the posterior cutaneous nerve of the thigh (S1,2,3).

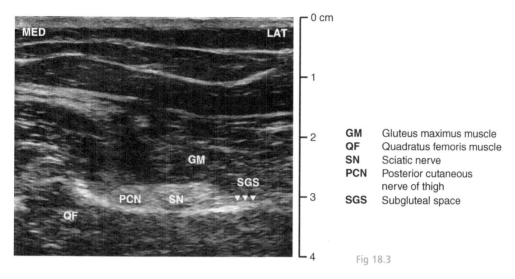

GM	Gluteus maximus muscle
QF	Quadratus femoris muscle
SN	Sciatic nerve
PCN	Posterior cutaneous nerve of thigh
SGS	Subgluteal space

Fig 18.3

Diagram of scan

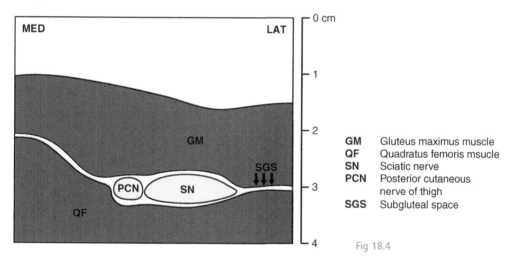

GM	Gluteus maximus muscle
QF	Quadratus femoris msucle
SN	Sciatic nerve
PCN	Posterior cutaneous nerve of thigh
SGS	Subgluteal space

Fig 18.4

Tips and complications Using in-plane insertion of the needle helps the operator to avoid nerve penetration. Local anaesthetic spread can be observed directly, dilating the subgluteal space, and ensuring even spread around the nerve.

Damage to the sciatic nerve may follow multiple punctures of the nerve or failure to use an atraumatic short-bevel needle.

In spite of its size, the sciatic nerve can be difficult to visualize because of its depth, 3–5 cm, and due to anisotropy. This applies particularly when a linear probe is used. In such a case:

- Use a curvilinear probe, which may enable simultaneous visualization of the bony landmarks of the ischial tuberosity and greater trochanter. This makes identification of the subgluteal space easier.
- Track the sciatic nerve proximally from the popliteal fossa, where it can be easily picked up just deep to biceps femoris and lateral to the popliteal vessels.
- Tilt the probe to adjust for anisotropy.

Anatomy of the tibial nerve in the popliteal fossa

The sciatic nerve (L4,5, S1,2,3) descends in the posterior aspect of the thigh, passing distally from the gluteal region to the popliteal fossa. It lies in a space bounded medially by the semimembranosus and semitendinosus muscles, and is covered posterolaterally by the long head of the biceps femoris muscle. As the sciatic nerve enters the popliteal fossa it divides to form the tibial and common peroneal nerves, coming to lie deep to biceps femoris and lateral to the popliteal vessels.

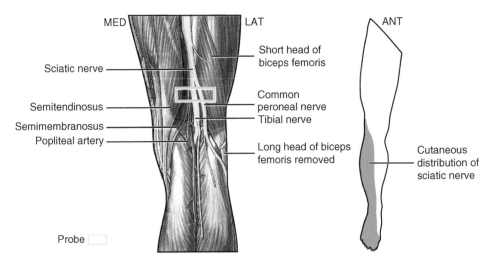

Fig 19.1

Probe placement for tibial nerve block in popliteal fossa

Identify the greater trochanter and the ischial tuberosity. A linear probe is then placed halfway between these landmarks over the popliteal pulse.

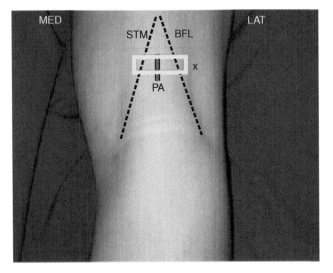

STM Semimembranosus and semitendinosus
BFL Biceps femoris (long head)
PA Popliteal artery
X Needle entry point

Probe

Fig 19.2

Scan of tibial nerve in popliteal fossa

At this level the tibial nerve lies between the semimembranosus (and semitendinosus) muscles and the biceps femoris muscle (long and short heads). It usually lies beneath the medial edge of the long head of biceps femoris. Lateral to the tibial nerve can be seen the common peroneal nerve.

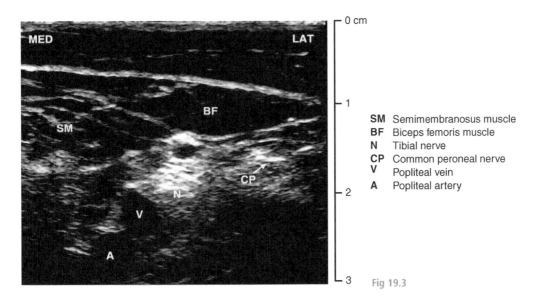

SM Semimembranosus muscle
BF Biceps femoris muscle
N   Tibial nerve
CP Common peroneal nerve
V   Popliteal vein
A   Popliteal artery

Fig 19.3

Diagram of scan

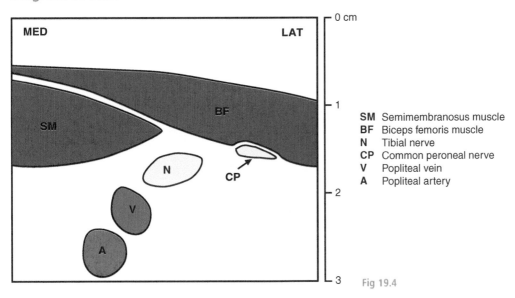

SM Semimembranosus muscle
BF Biceps femoris muscle
N   Tibial nerve
CP Common peroneal nerve
V   Popliteal vein
A   Popliteal artery

Fig 19.4

Tips and complications Needle insertion is performed in plane, approaching from the lateral aspect in order to avoid the popliteal vessels. The main complication is puncture of the popliteal vessels.

Anatomy of the posterior cutaneous nerve of the thigh

The posterior cutaneous nerve of the thigh (PCNT) is formed from the anterior rami of S1,2,3 in the sacral plexus. It has the largest cutaneous distribution of all the cutaneous nerves covering the lower buttock, lateral perineum, posterior thigh and popliteal fossa. It accompanies the sciatic nerve into the posterior thigh, becoming subcutaneous at the lower border of gluteus maximus.

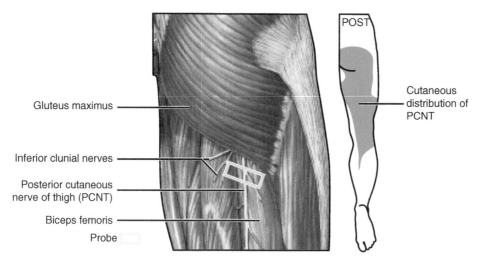

Fig 20.1

Probe placement for block of posterior cutaneous nerve of thigh

Locate the inferior margin of gluteus maximus at the level of the greater trochanter. Identify the biceps femoris muscle, the lateral hamstring, by getting the patient to flex the knee against resistance. The probe is placed across biceps femoris.

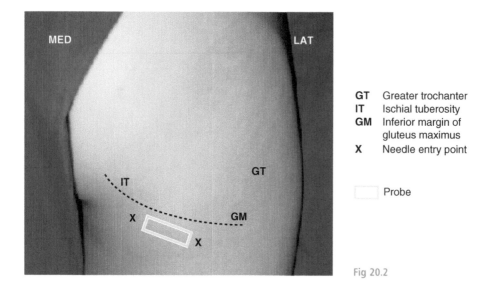

GT Greater trochanter
IT Ischial tuberosity
GM Inferior margin of gluteus maximus
X Needle entry point

Probe

Fig 20.2

Scan of posterior cutaneous nerve of thigh

The PCNT is subcutaneous and located on the surface of biceps femoris. Increasing the depth of the scan will reveal the sciatic nerve deep to biceps femoris.

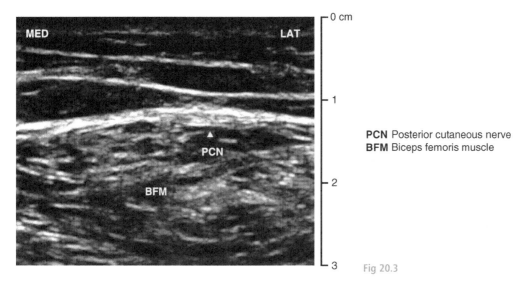

PCN Posterior cutaneous nerve
BFM Biceps femoris muscle

Fig 20.3

Diagram of scan

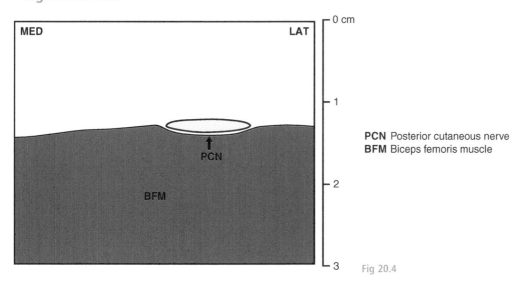

PCN Posterior cutaneous nerve
BFM Biceps femoris muscle

Fig 20.4

Tips and complications The PCNT is a peripheral nerve which is not easily visualized. A simple block can be obtained by passing the needle through the biceps femoris fascia and injecting into the biceps femoris compartment. A stimulator can be used to confirm identity of the PCNT and locate the electrode close to the nerve for radiofrequency lesioning.

Anatomy of the common peroneal nerve

The common peroneal (fibular) nerve (L4,5, S1,2) is formed from the sciatic nerve as it enters the apex of the popliteal fossa. It supplies the muscles of the anterior compartment of the lower leg (injury resulting in 'drop foot') and the skin of the anterolateral aspect of the lower leg, extending over the dorsum of the foot. It passes behind the knee along the medial border of biceps femoris (long head) to run behind the head of the fibula, where it splits into deep peroneal and superficial peroneal branches.

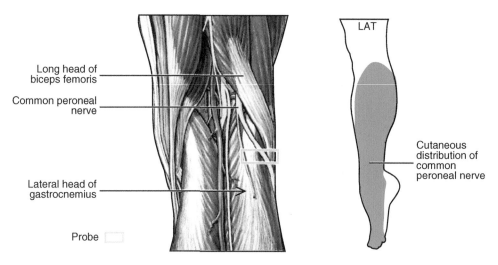

Fig 21.1

Probe placement for common peroneal nerve block

Identify the long head of the biceps femoris muscle, which forms the lower lateral border of the popliteal fossa at the level of the head of fibula. Place a linear probe across the space between biceps femoris and the lateral head of gastrocnemius.

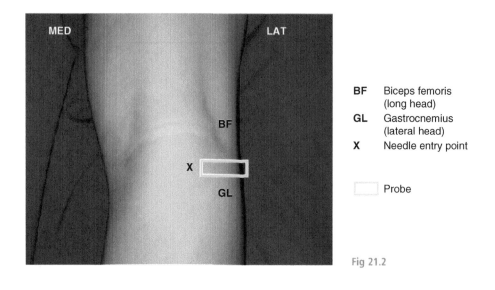

BF   Biceps femoris (long head)

GL   Gastrocnemius (lateral head)

X   Needle entry point

    Probe

Fig 21.2

Scan of common peroneal nerve

At the level of the fibular head, the common peroneal nerve is superficial and related to the medial edge of the long head of biceps femoris. It lies on the surface of gastrocnemius (lateral head).

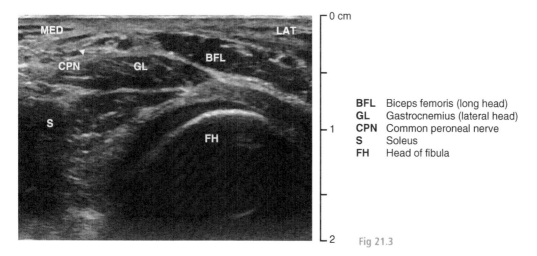

BFL Biceps femoris (long head)
GL Gastrocnemius (lateral head)
CPN Common peroneal nerve
S Soleus
FH Head of fibula

Fig 21.3

Diagram of scan

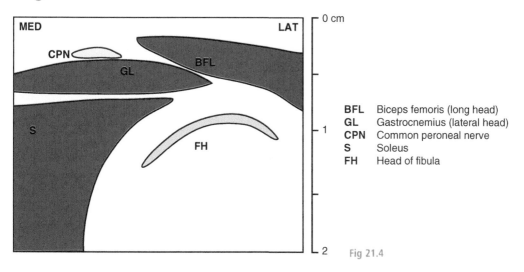

BFL Biceps femoris (long head)
GL Gastrocnemius (lateral head)
CPN Common peroneal nerve
S Soleus
FH Head of fibula

Fig 21.4

Tips and complications Identify the common peroneal nerve at its formation from the sciatic nerve at the apex of the popliteal fossa, where the sciatic nerve divides to form the tibial and common peroneal nerves. Track the common peroneal nerve distally to the fibular head. Needle insertion is performed in plane, approaching from the lateral aspect in order to avoid the popliteal vessels. Puncture of the popliteal vessels is a possible complication.

Anatomy of the saphenous nerve in the lower leg

The saphenous nerve in the lower leg is a terminal cutaneous branch of the femoral nerve and takes its origin from L3,4, supplying an area over the medial aspect of the lower leg, ankle and foot. It passes to the lower leg in the adductor canal between the sartorius and gracilis muscles, emerging subcutaneously just above the knee.

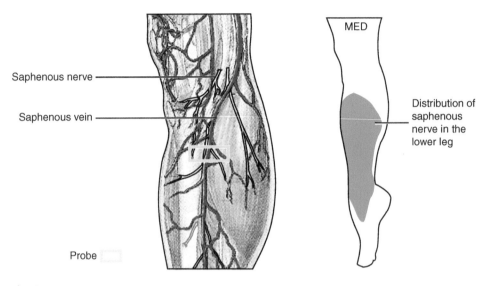

Saphenous nerve

Saphenous vein

Probe

MED

Distribution of saphenous nerve in the lower leg

Fig 22.1

Probe placement for saphenous nerve block in lower leg

Place a linear probe over the medial aspect of the lower leg, just below the knee joint, with the anterior end of the probe over the posterior border of the tibia.

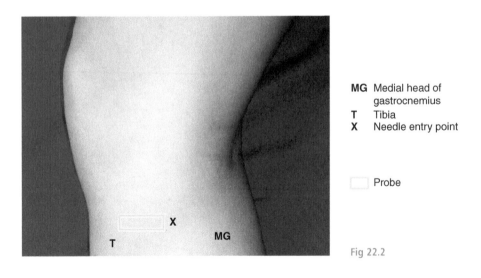

MG Medial head of gastrocnemius
T Tibia
X Needle entry point

Probe

Fig 22.2

Scan of saphenous nerve in lower leg

The landmarks in this scan are the tibia and its drop-out shadow in the bottom left hand corner, and the saphenous vein, which is superficial. The saphenous nerve lies close to the vein and may be divided at this point.

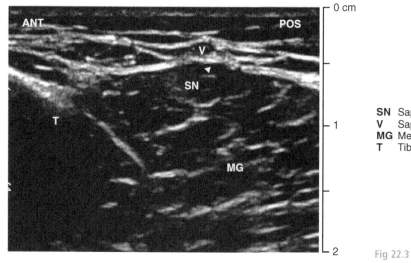

SN   Saphenous nerve
V   Saphenous vein
MG   Medial gastrocnemius
T   Tibia and drop-out shadow

Fig 22.3

Diagram of scan

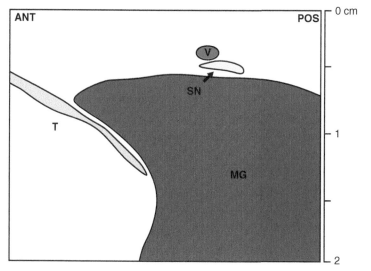

SN   Saphenous nerve
V   Saphenous vein
MG   Medial gastrocnemius
T   Tibia and drop-out shadow

Fig 22.4

Tips and complications Use a nerve stimulator to identify the nerve for neurolytic lesioning.

Anatomy of the sural nerve in the calf

The sural nerve (S1,2) is a cutaneous nerve arising from the tibial nerve and a communicating branch from the common popliteal nerve. It is the sensory supply to the lateral aspect of the heel and mid foot as well as a posterolateral area of the lower calf. The sural nerve is formed in the popliteal fossa and descends between the heads of gastrocnemius to become superficial in the mid calf. It is accompanied by and lies lateral to the small saphenous vein.

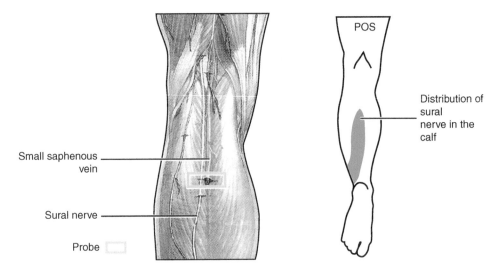

Fig 23.1

Probe placement for sural nerve block in calf

With the patient in the lateral or prone position, use a linear probe placed transversely across the groove between the medial and lateral heads of gastrocnemius, at mid calf level.

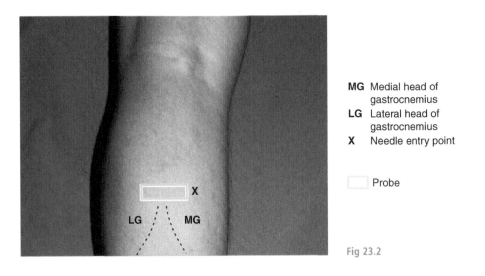

MG Medial head of gastrocnemius
LG Lateral head of gastrocnemius
X Needle entry point

Probe

Fig 23.2

Scan of sural nerve in calf

The small saphenous vein is a useful vascular landmark, the sural nerve usually lying lateral to this small subcutaneous vessel.

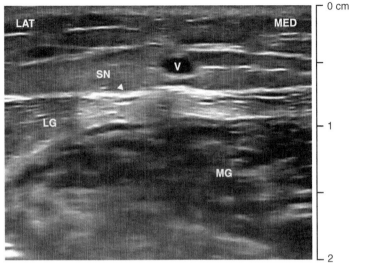

V Small saphenous vein
MG Medial gastrocnemius
LG Lateral gastrocnemius
SN Sural nerve

Fig 23.3

Diagram of scan

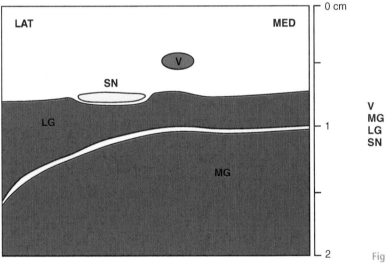

V Small saphenous vein
MG Medial gastrocnemius
LG Lateral gastrocnemius
SN Sural nerve

Fig 23.4

Tips and complications Insert needle out of plane, and confirm identity and proximity of the needle tip for radiofrequency lesioning with nerve stimulator. The only complication is puncture of small saphenous vein.

Anatomy of the posterior tibial nerve in the lower leg

The posterior tibial nerve (PTN) (L5, S1,2,3) is the terminal branch of the sciatic nerve supplying the intrinsic muscles of the foot and sensation to the sole of the foot and the heel. In the lower leg above the medial malleolus, it gives off calcaneal branches before reaching the ankle. The nerve accompanies the posterior tibial artery and the accompanying veins, lying deep (lateral) to the vessels. In the ankle this nerve splits into medial plantar and lateral plantar branches. Block the nerve in the lower leg if cover of calcaneal branches is required.

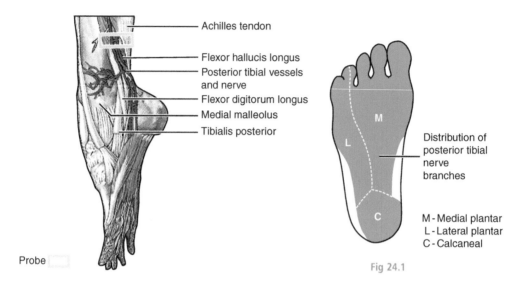

— Achilles tendon

— Flexor hallucis longus
— Posterior tibial vessels and nerve
— Flexor digitorum longus
— Medial malleolus
— Tibialis posterior

M
L
C

Distribution of posterior tibial nerve branches

M - Medial plantar
L - Lateral plantar
C - Calcaneal

Probe

Fig 24.1

Probe placement for posterior tibial nerve block in lower leg

Use a small linear probe and place it transversely across the space between the tibia and the Achilles tendon, 2–4 cm above the medial malleolus.

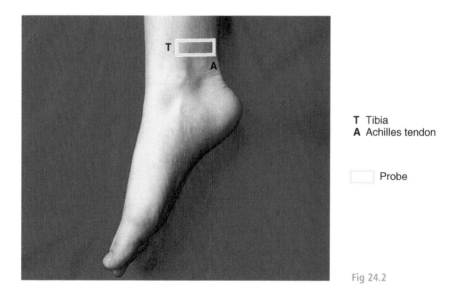

T Tibia
A Achilles tendon

Probe

Fig 24.2

Scan of posterior tibial nerve in lower leg

The landmarks used in this scan are vascular (posterior tibial vessels) and bony (the tibia). The posterior tibial nerve can be seen deep to the vessels. In this scan it has given off a calcaneal branch.

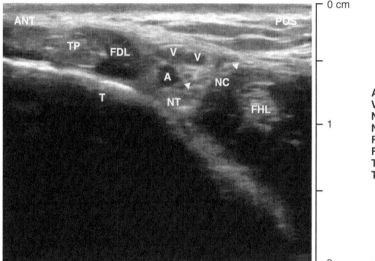

A   Posterior tibial artery
V   Posterior tibial vein
NT Posterior tibial nerve
NC Calcaneal branch
FDL Flexor digitorum longus tendon
FHL Flexor hallucis longus tendon
TP Tibialis posterior tendon
T   Tibia

Fig 24.3

Diagram of scan

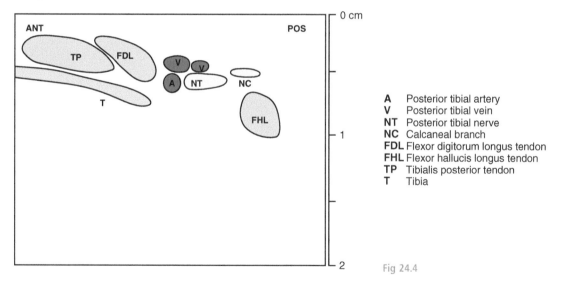

A   Posterior tibial artery
V   Posterior tibial vein
NT Posterior tibial nerve
NC Calcaneal branch
FDL Flexor digitorum longus tendon
FHL Flexor hallucis longus tendon
TP Tibialis posterior tendon
T   Tibia

Fig 24.4

Tips and complications Insert the needle in plane from the posterior aspect of the probe, as the tibia tends to obstruct the anterior approach and also makes the angle of insertion steeper, reducing visibility of the needle. Damage to the posterior tibial vessels can occur as a complication.

Anatomy of the deep peroneal nerve

The common peroneal nerve splits to form the deep peroneal nerve (DPN) and the superficial peroneal nerve (SPN) as it passes between fibularis longus and the neck of the fibula in the lateral compartment of the lower leg. As the DPN descends in the lower leg it lies deep on the interosseous membrane and enters the dorsum of the foot, lying lateral to the extensor hallucis longus tendon and the dorsalis pedis artery.

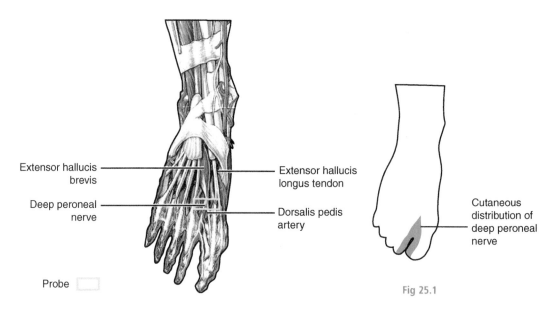

Extensor hallucis brevis

Deep peroneal nerve

Probe

Extensor hallucis longus tendon

Dorsalis pedis artery

Cutaneous distribution of deep peroneal nerve

Fig 25.1

Probe placement for deep peroneal nerve block

Place the probe transversely across the dorsalis pedis artery and extensor hallucis longus tendon on the dorsum of the foot.

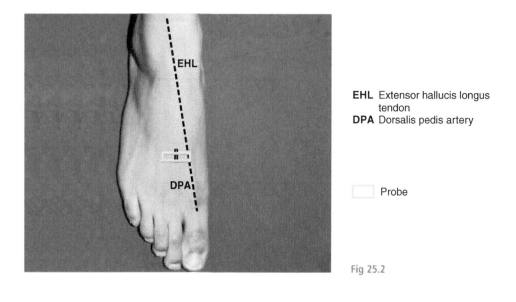

EHL Extensor hallucis longus tendon
DPA Dorsalis pedis artery

Probe

Fig 25.2

Scan of deep peroneal nerve

The main landmark in this scan is the dorsalis pedis artery. The DPN may lie to either side of the artery, but is usually found medial to the extensor hallucis longus tendon. Inject both sides of the dorsalis pedis artery to block the deep peroneal nerve.

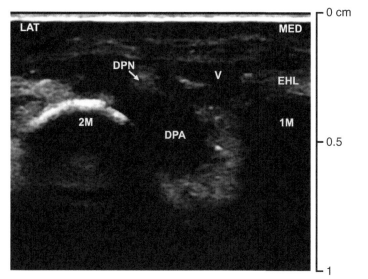

EHL   Extensor hallucis longus
DPN   Deep peroneal nerve
DPA   Dorsalis pedis artery
V   Vein
2M   2nd metatarsal
1M   1st metatarsal

Fig 25.3

Diagram of scan

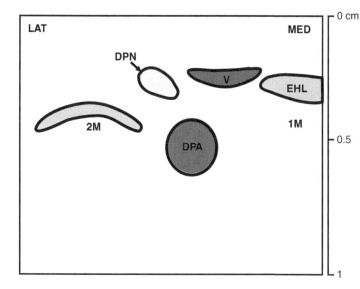

EHL   Extensor hallucis longus
DPN   Deep peroneal nerve
DPA   Dorsalis pedis artery
V   Vein
2M   2nd metatarsal
1M   1st metatarsal

Fig 25.4

Tips and complications Use a small linear probe to bridge the gap between the first and second metatarsals. The main landmark is the dorsalis pedis artery. The deep peroneal is usually lateral to the artery. Puncture of the dorsalis pedis artery may occur as a complication.

61

Anatomy of the superficial peroneal nerve

The superficial peroneal nerve (SPN) is formed from the common peroneal nerve as it enters the lateral compartment of the lower leg, at the level of the fibular head. The SPN passes distally in the lateral compartment and pierces the deep fascia to become subcutaneous in the distal third of the leg. Its branches supply the skin over the dorsum of the foot and toes apart from a small area between the big toe and second toe (supplied by the deep peroneal nerve) and the lateral aspect of the little toe.

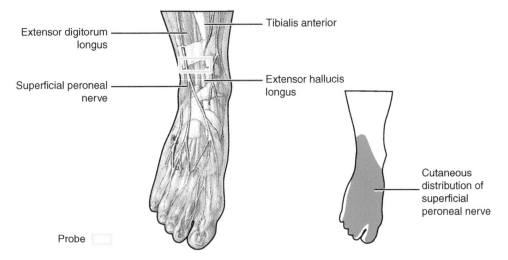

Extensor digitorum longus

Tibialis anterior

Superficial peroneal nerve

Extensor hallucis longus

Cutaneous distribution of superficial peroneal nerve

Probe

Fig 26.1

Probe placement for superficial peroneal nerve block

Place the probe transversely across the extensor digitorum longus (EDL) muscle and extensor hallucis longus (EHL) tendon, at the level of the medial and lateral malleoli.

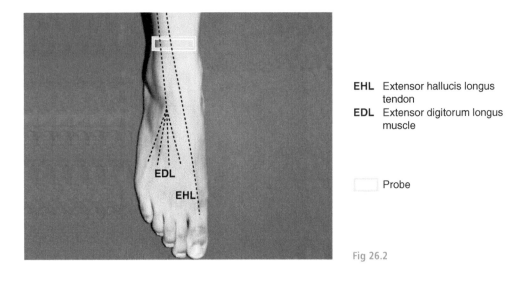

EHL Extensor hallucis longus tendon
EDL Extensor digitorum longus muscle

☐ Probe

EDL
EHL

Fig 26.2

Scan of superficial peroneal nerve

The anterior surface of the tibia forms the bottom of the scan, with the anterior tibial artery and deep peroneal nerve resting on it. The muscle running across the tibial surface is EDL, and the SPN lies on its surface in the subcutaneous layer.

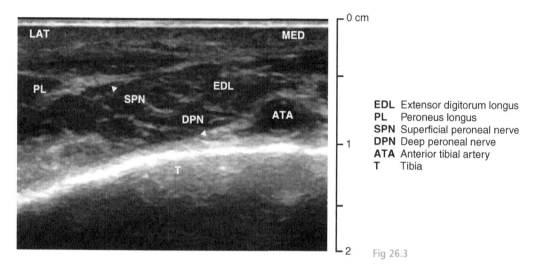

EDL Extensor digitorum longus
PL   Peroneus longus
SPN Superficial peroneal nerve
DPN Deep peroneal nerve
ATA Anterior tibial artery
T   Tibia

Fig 26.3

Diagram of scan

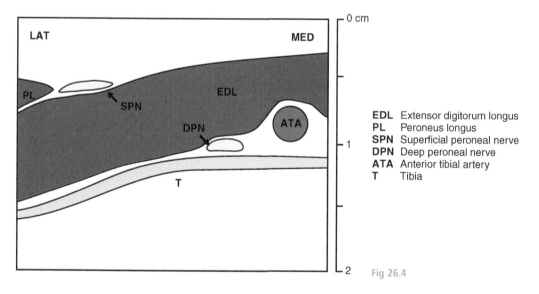

EDL Extensor digitorum longus
PL   Peroneus longus
SPN Superficial peroneal nerve
DPN Deep peroneal nerve
ATA Anterior tibial artery
T   Tibia

Fig 26.4

Tips and complications Identify EDL and EHL muscles by asking the patient to extend his or her toes and big toe. Puncture of the anterior tibial artery is a complication.

Anatomy of the saphenous nerve in the thigh

The saphenous nerve in the thigh is a terminal cutaneous branch of the femoral nerve and takes its origin from L3,4. It supplies an area over the medial aspect of the knee, lower leg and foot. It passes to the lower leg in the adductor canal between the sartorius and gracilis muscles, emerging subcutaneously just below the knee.

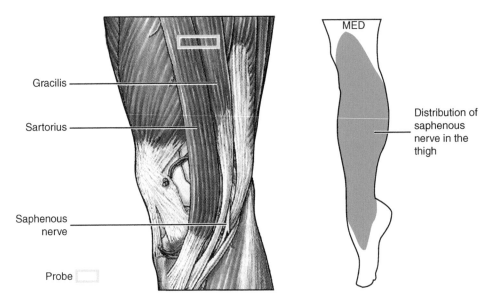

Gracilis

Sartorius

Saphenous nerve

Probe

MED

Distribution of saphenous nerve in the thigh

Fig 27.1

Probe placement for saphenous nerve block in thigh

Place a linear probe over the medial aspect of the thigh, above the knee joint, with the probe across the posterior border of the sartorius muscle.

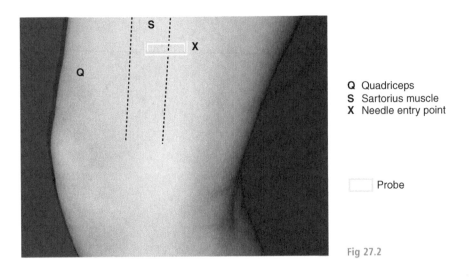

Q Quadriceps
S Sartorius muscle
X Needle entry point

Probe

Fig 27.2

Scan of saphenous nerve in thigh

The landmarks in this scan are the sartorius and gracilis muscles. Deep to the posterior border of sartorius in the space between sartorius and gracilis lies the saphenous nerve, usually accompanied by a small vein.

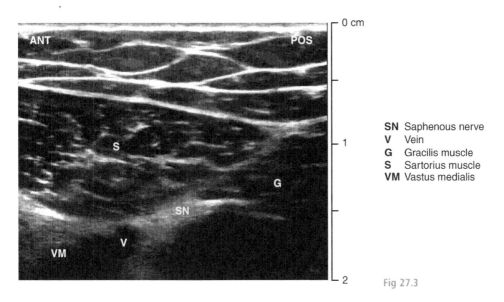

SN Saphenous nerve
V Vein
G Gracilis muscle
S Sartorius muscle
VM Vastus medialis

Fig 27.3

Diagram of scan

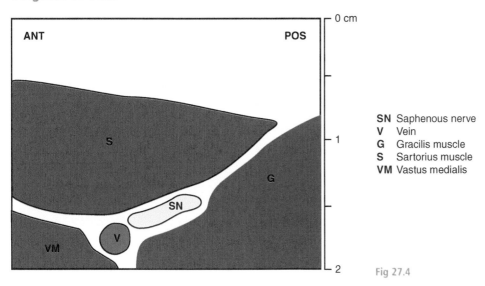

SN Saphenous nerve
V Vein
G Gracilis muscle
S Sartorius muscle
VM Vastus medialis

Fig 27.4

Tips and complications Track the sartorius muscle distally from the anterior thigh, where the anterior border of sartorius forms the lateral margin of the femoral triangle.

Anatomy of the sural nerve in the lower leg

The sural nerve (L5, S1) is a sensory nerve formed by branches from the tibial nerve and the common peroneal nerve. It passes subcutaneously from the mid calf into the ankle and foot, accompanying the small saphenous vein, lying lateral to the Achilles tendon as it passes distally to the foot. At the ankle the sural nerve forms lateral calcaneal and lateral dorsal terminal branches.

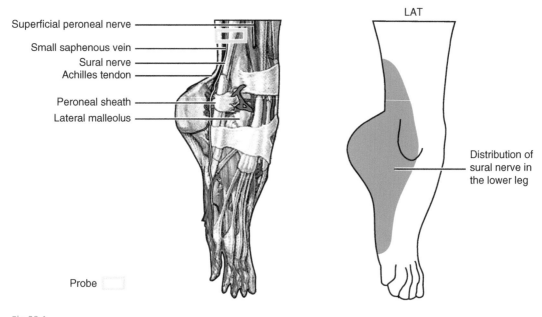

Superficial peroneal nerve
Small saphenous vein
Sural nerve
Achilles tendon
Peroneal sheath
Lateral malleolus

Probe

LAT

Distribution of sural nerve in the lower leg

Fig 28.1

Probe placement for sural nerve block in lower leg

In this approach to the sural nerve, a linear probe is placed transversely across the space between the fibula and the Achilles tendon, at a level 2–4 cm above the lateral malleolus.

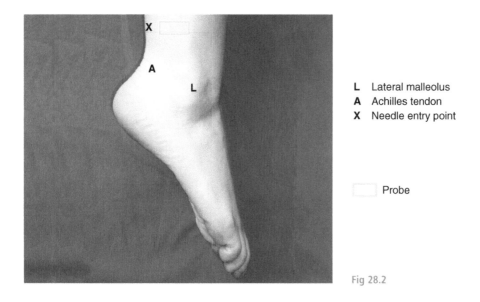

X
A
L

L   Lateral malleolus
A   Achilles tendon
X   Needle entry point

Probe

Fig 28.2

Scan of sural nerve in lower leg

The bony landmark in this scan is the fibula on the right side. Two tendons of peroneus longus and peroneus brevis are immediately posterior to the lateral malleolus, and can be identified by asking the patient to evert the foot. Posterior and superficial to these tendons in their sheath is the sural nerve, accompanied by the small saphenous vein.

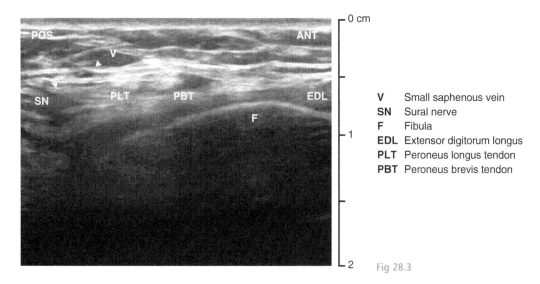

V	Small saphenous vein
SN	Sural nerve
F	Fibula
EDL	Extensor digitorum longus
PLT	Peroneus longus tendon
PBT	Peroneus brevis tendon

Fig 28.3

Diagram of scan

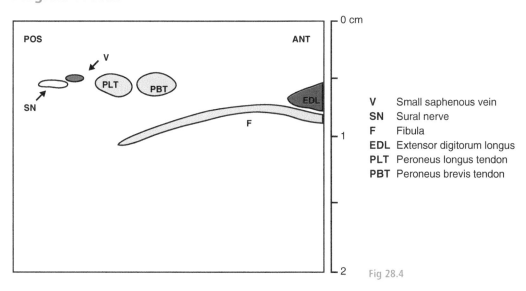

V	Small saphenous vein
SN	Sural nerve
F	Fibula
EDL	Extensor digitorum longus
PLT	Peroneus longus tendon
PBT	Peroneus brevis tendon

Fig 28.4

Tips and complications Insert the needle in plane from the posterior aspect of the probe, as the fibula may obstruct the anterior approach. The nerve is subcutaneous.

Anatomy of the posterior tibial nerve at the ankle

The posterior tibial nerve (PTN) (L5, S1,2,3) is the terminal branch of the sciatic nerve supplying the intrinsic muscles of the foot and sensation to the sole of the foot and the heel. In the ankle it is found in the space between the medial malleolus and the Achilles tendon. The PTN runs deep (lateral) to the posterior tibial artery and its accompanying veins. Before entering the ankle, PTN gives off a medial branch to the calcaneus. Blocking the nerve in the ankle may miss this calcaneal branch. In the ankle PTN splits into medial plantar and lateral plantar branches.

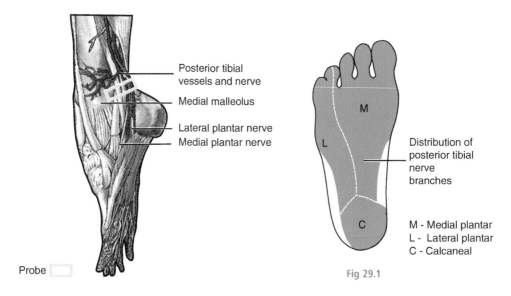

Posterior tibial vessels and nerve

Medial malleolus

Lateral plantar nerve
Medial plantar nerve

M

L

Distribution of posterior tibial nerve branches

C

M - Medial plantar
L - Lateral plantar
C - Calcaneal

Probe

Fig 29.1

Probe placement for posterior tibial nerve block at ankle

Use a small linear probe (or hockey stick probe) and place it transversely across the space between the medial malleolus and the Achilles tendon.

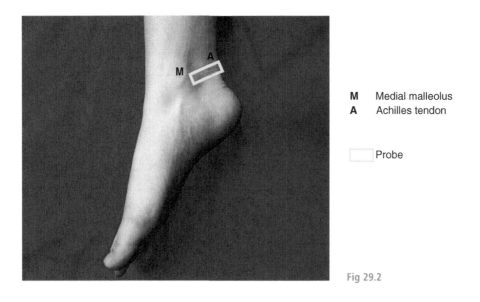

M   Medial malleolus
A   Achilles tendon

Probe

Fig 29.2

Scan of posterior tibial nerve at ankle

The landmarks used in this scan are vascular (posterior tibial artery with accompanying veins) and bony (medial malleolus). The posterior tibial nerve can be seen deep to the posterior tibial vessels. In this scan the posterior tibial nerve is dividing into its terminal lateral and medial plantar branches.

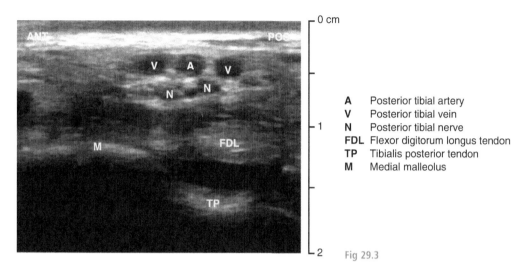

A	Posterior tibial artery
V	Posterior tibial vein
N	Posterior tibial nerve
FDL	Flexor digitorum longus tendon
TP	Tibialis posterior tendon
M	Medial malleolus

Fig 29.3

Diagram of scan

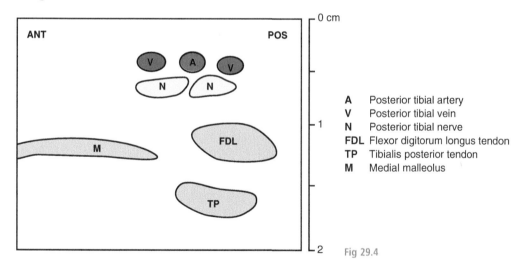

A	Posterior tibial artery
V	Posterior tibial vein
N	Posterior tibial nerve
FDL	Flexor digitorum longus tendon
TP	Tibialis posterior tendon
M	Medial malleolus

Fig 29.4

Tips and complications Insert the needle in plane from the posterior aspect of the probe, as the medial malleolus tends to obstruct the anterior approach and also makes the angle of insertion steeper, thus reducing visibility of the needle. Damage to the posterior tibial vessels can occur as a complication. Blocking the posterior tibial nerve in the ankle may miss the calcaneal branch, therefore block the nerve in the lower leg for coverage of the heel (see *posterior tibial nerve in the lower leg*).

69

Anatomy of the sural nerve at the ankle

The sural nerve (L5, S1) is a sensory nerve formed by branches from the tibial nerve and the common peroneal nerve. These branches give rise to the sural nerve subcutaneously at the junction of the heads of gastrocnemius in the calf (see *sural nerve in the calf*). The sural nerve accompanies the small saphenous vein, lying lateral to the Achilles tendon as it passes distally to the foot. At the ankle the sural nerve forms lateral calcaneal and lateral dorsal terminal branches.

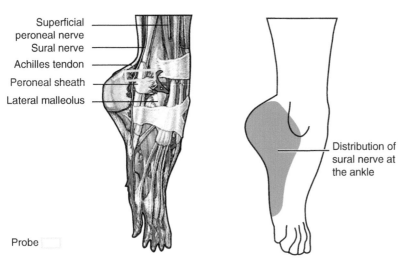

Superficial peroneal nerve
Sural nerve
Achilles tendon
Peroneal sheath
Lateral malleolus

Distribution of sural nerve at the ankle

Probe

Fig 30.1

Probe placement for sural nerve block at ankle

Use a small linear probe and place it transversely across the space between the lateral malleolus and the Achilles tendon.

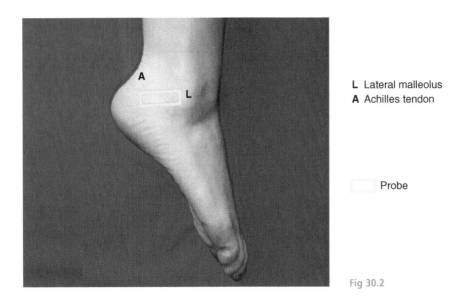

L Lateral malleolus
A Achilles tendon

Probe

Fig 30.2

Scan of sural nerve at ankle

This scan bridges the space between the two bony landmarks of the lateral malleolus with its drop-out shadow, and the lateral surface of the calcaneum. Two tendons of peroneus longus and peroneus brevis are immediately posterior to the lateral malleolus, and can be identified by asking the patient to evert the foot. These tendons are enclosed by the peroneal sheath. The sural nerve is a small subcutaneous nerve outside the sheath.

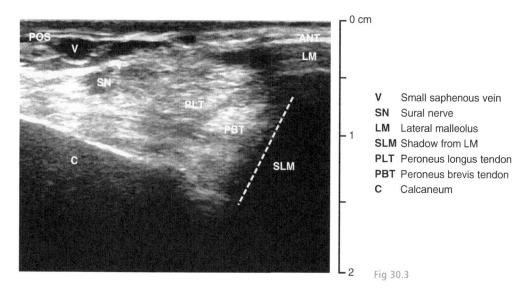

V	Small saphenous vein
SN	Sural nerve
LM	Lateral malleolus
SLM	Shadow from LM
PLT	Peroneus longus tendon
PBT	Peroneus brevis tendon
C	Calcaneum

Fig 30.3

Diagram of scan

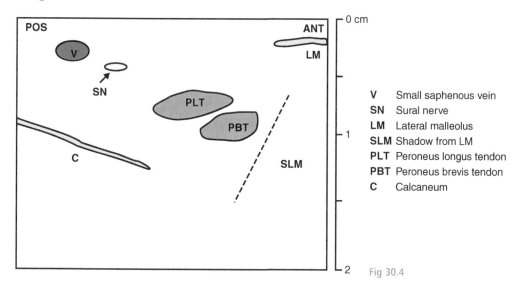

V	Small saphenous vein
SN	Sural nerve
LM	Lateral malleolus
SLM	Shadow from LM
PLT	Peroneus longus tendon
PBT	Peroneus brevis tendon
C	Calcaneum

Fig 30.4

Tips and complications Use a small linear or hockey-stick probe, because the medial malleolus may get in the way. Insert the needle in plane from the postero-inferior aspect of the probe, as the lateral malleolus tends to obstruct the anterior approach. This is a peripheral block with no major complications.

The lumbar spine

The main features in the sonoanatomy of the spine are the bony profiles seen in the ultrasound scans. Using these profiles, bony features such as the articular processes forming the facet joints can be identified. It is also possible to visualize soft tissue structures such as the ligamentum flavum and dorsal dura, which appear as a single layer, the ligamentum flavum/dorsal dura complex (LFD). Ultrasound can then be used to prescan and find the best needle entry point and trajectory, or to guide injections in real time.

Median plane

Longitudinal views are not usually taken in the median plane (mid-line) because the 'drop-out shadows' of the vertebral spines tends to obscure tissue penetration in the intervertebral spaces. This is due to their shape (the tip of the spine being wider than the base) and their caudad angulation, both features causing the spine to overshadow the intervertebral space below.

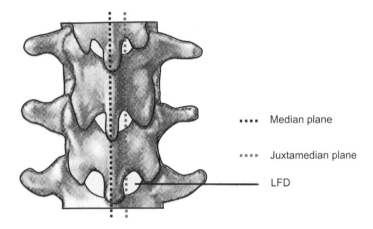

•••• Median plane

•••• Juxtamedian plane

——— LFD

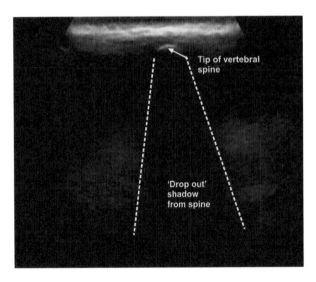

Fig 31.1 **Dorsal view of lumbar spine and longitudinal scan in median plane**

Juxtamedian plane

Scanning longitudinally in a plane just next to the median plane, but angled slightly towards the midline, is performed in order to obtain improved views of the soft tissues in the intervertebral space. In particular, good visualization of the ligamentum flavum/dorsal dura complex (LFD) can be achieved. This plane is referred to as the *juxtamedian* plane and is illustrated in Figure 31.2.

In the juxtamedian plane reflections of the ultrasound beam are obtained from the base of the vertebral spine, the lamina and the LFD. In the juxtamedian scan these reflections appear as a series of '3 steps'. A fourth fainter reflection can often be seen, as in the bottom left-hand corner of the scan: this is from the ventral dura or vertebral body.

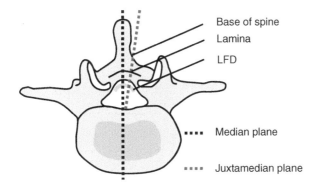

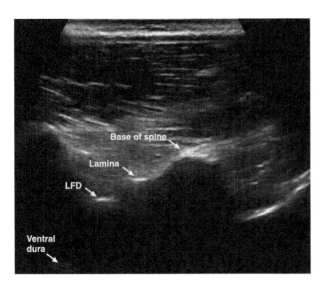

Fig 31.2 **Juxtamedian plane in cross-section and longitudinal scan in juxtamedian plane**

Lumbosacral junction

A convenient landmark when scanning the lumbar spine is the lumbosacral junction (Fig. 31.3). This is readily identifiable on scanning in the juxtamedian plane, and acts as a reference point from which the intervertebral spaces can be accurately numbered.

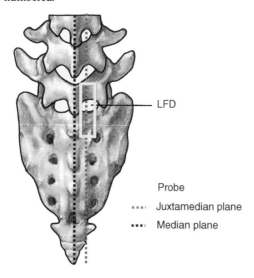

LFD

Probe

···· Juxtamedian plane

···· Median plane

Fig 31.3 **Dorsal view of the lumbosacral junction**

Probe placement over the lumbosacral junction

Start with a curvilinear probe over the sacrum and move cephalad to the lumbosacral junction. Then move laterally into the juxtamedian plane, remembering to keep the probe tilted towards the midline.

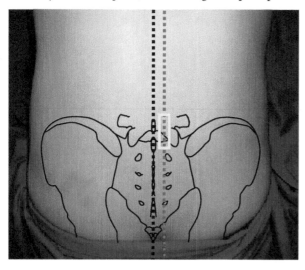

Fig 31.4 **Probe placement for juxtamedian view of lumbosacral junction**

Juxtamedian scan of lumbosacral junction

In this scan the sacrum is first identified in the midline by the continuous bony profile produced by reflection from the median crest of the sacrum. On moving the probe cephalad in the midline, this continuous profile gives way to an interrupted reflection from the tips of the vertebral spines. The probe can then be moved laterally into the juxtamedian plane at the lumbosacral junction in order to view the ligamentum flavum/dorsal dura layer (LFD) in the L5–S1 intervertebral space.

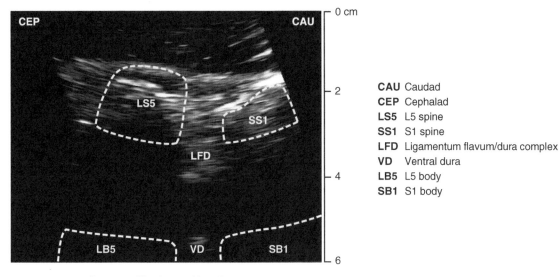

CAU	Caudad
CEP	Cephalad
LS5	L5 spine
SS1	S1 spine
LFD	Ligamentum flavum/dura complex
VD	Ventral dura
LB5	L5 body
SB1	S1 body

Fig 31.5 **Juxtamedian scan of lumbosacral junction**

Diagram of scan

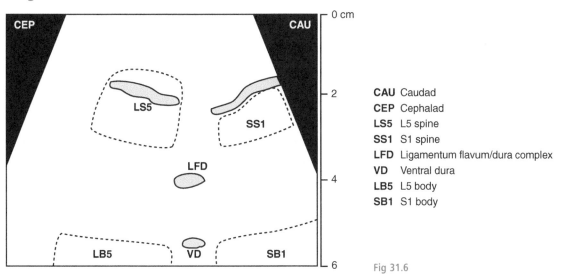

CAU	Caudad
CEP	Cephalad
LS5	L5 spine
SS1	S1 spine
LFD	Ligamentum flavum/dura complex
VD	Ventral dura
LB5	L5 body
SB1	S1 body

Fig 31.6

75

L3–L4 intervertebral space

The appearance of a juxtamedian scan of the lumbar spine is best understood by examining a midline section of the vertebra at L3 and L4. The juxtamedian plane is described above; in Fig. 31.6, the ultrasound beam is angled from the far side of the vertebral spines towards the reader. The beam will strike the far side of the vertebral spines at the broken red lines (producing reflections) and pass through the interspinous gap to produce reflections from the lamina, the ligamentum flavum/dorsal dura complex (LFD) and the ventral dura (solid red lines). Thus the reflections in a juxtamedian scan are produced by the bases of the spines, the lamina, the LFD and the ventral dura.

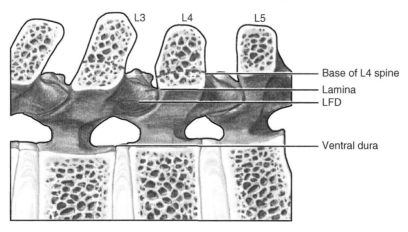

Fig 31.7 **Longitudinal section at L3–L4**

Probe placement over L3–L4 intervertebral space

Identify the juxtamedian plane, by finding the line of the median plane and moving the probe just laterally, while keeping the probe tilted towards the midline. Starting at the lumbosacral junction, count intervertebral spaces in a cepahalad direction until the L3–L4 space can be identified.

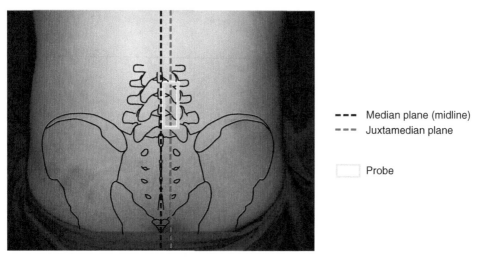

Fig 31.8 **Probe placement for juxtamedian scan at L3–L4**

Juxtamedian scan of L3–L4 intervertebral space

In this juxtamedian scan of the lumbar spine the positions of the vertebral spines and bodies of L3 and L4 are indicated by the broken yellow outlines. The reflections in the scan (labelled LS4, L and LFD) correspond to the features labelled in Fig. 31.7 with solid and broken red lines. These reflections from the base of the spine, the lamina and the LFD can be loosely visualized as a shape of three shallow 'steps'.

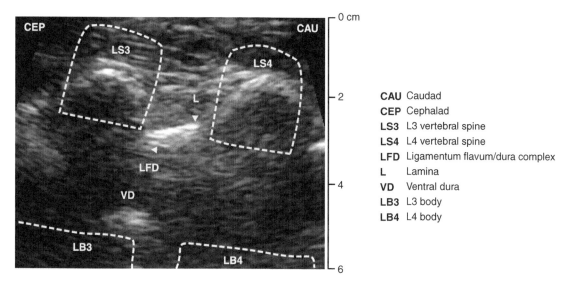

Fig 31.9 **Juxtamedian scan at L3–L4**

CAU	Caudad
CEP	Cephalad
LS3	L3 vertebral spine
LS4	L4 vertebral spine
LFD	Ligamentum flavum/dura complex
L	Lamina
VD	Ventral dura
LB3	L3 body
LB4	L4 body

Diagram of scan

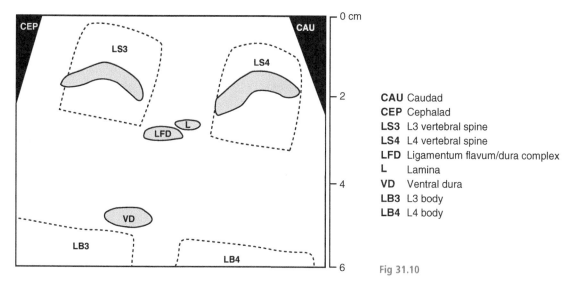

CAU	Caudad
CEP	Cephalad
LS3	L3 vertebral spine
LS4	L4 vertebral spine
LFD	Ligamentum flavum/dura complex
L	Lamina
VD	Ventral dura
LB3	L3 body
LB4	L4 body

Fig 31.10

Longitudinal view of facet joints at L3 and L4

An ultrasound scan in a paramedian plane through the facet joints gives a characteristic appearance due to reflection from the bony profile of the articular processes. The typical appearance is a 'sawtooth' wave as shown by the red line in Fig. 31.10. The articular processes from adjacent vertebra form the facet joints, which maintain stability and alignment of the vertebra when they articulate with each other.

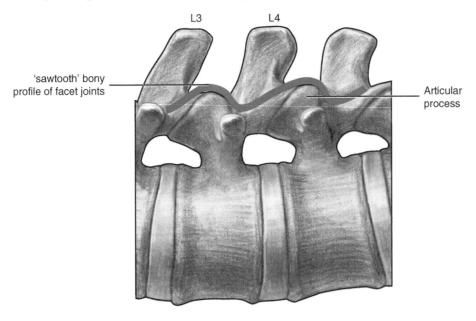

Fig 31.11 **Longitudinal view of facet joints at L3 and L4**

Probe placement for paramedian view of facet joints at L3 and L4

Count up to the L3–L4 intervertebral space from the lumbosacral junction in the juxtamedian plane. Move the probe laterally 1–2 cm until the typical 'sawtooth' profile appears in the scan.

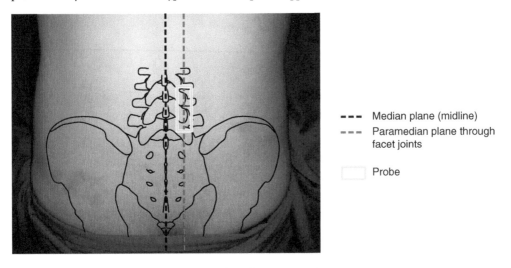

Fig 31.12 **Probe placement for paramedian view facet joints at L3 and L4**

Scan of lumbar facet joints at L3 and L4

This scan shows the characteristic 'sawtooth' profile of the facet joint between L3 and L4. In the facet joint between L3 and L4 (FJ34), both articular processes forming the joint can be identified. Periarticular injection can be performed in real time, using this view.

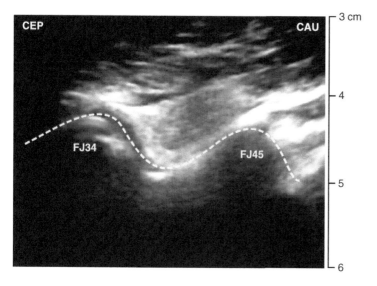

CAU Caudad
CEP Cephalad
FJ34 Facet joint between
      L3 and L4
FJ45 Facet joint between
      L4 and L5

Fig 31.13 **Scan of facet joints at L3 and L4**

Diagram of scan

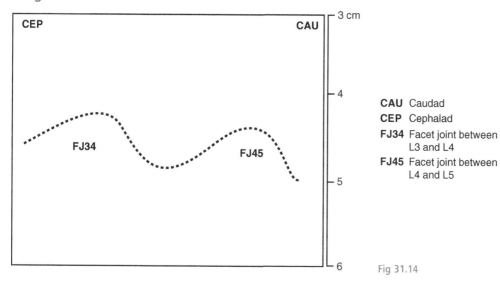

CAU Caudad
CEP Cephalad
FJ34 Facet joint between
      L3 and L4
FJ45 Facet joint between
      L4 and L5

Fig 31.14

Transverse view of L3–L4 intervertebral space

The ultrasound scan in a transverse plane at a lumbar intervertebral space will produce bright reflections and shadows according to the transverse bony profile of the vertebra. In Fig. 31.14 the position of the probe is shown, and the bony features of the vertebra producing 'bright' reflections in the scan are highlighted in red in the cross-section.

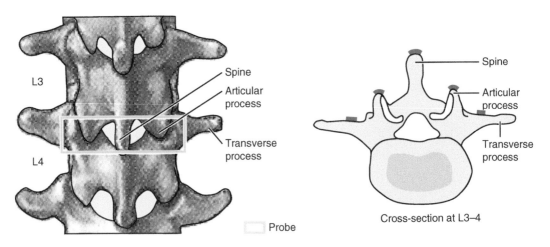

Cross-section at L3–4

Fig 31.15 **Transverse view in an intervertebral space (L3–L4)**

Probe placement for transverse view of L3–L4 intervertebral space

Start at the lumbosacral junction and locate the selected space (L3–L4) by counting in a cephalad direction, before rotating the probe into a transverse plane.

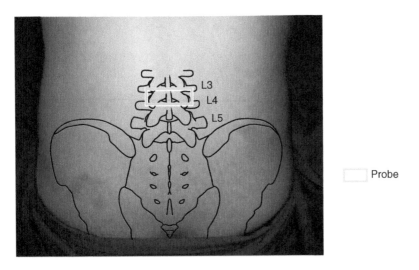

Fig 31.16 **Probe placement for transverse scan at L3–L4**

Transverse scan of L3–L4 intervertebral space

This transverse scan is taken between L3 and L4, and is tilted in a cephalad direction in order to avoid the vertebral spine and its drop-out shadow, which would otherwise obscure the view of the intervertebral space. Using this view the LFD can be visualized and its depth (d) measured. Note that while the drop-out shadow of the spine and the facet joint reflections are from L3, the reflections from the transverse processes are from L4.

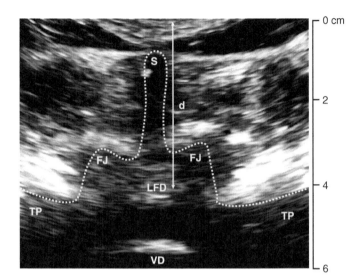

S	Vertebral spine
FJ	Facet joints
TP	Transverse processes
LFD	Ligamentum flavum/dura complex
VD	Ventral dura
d	Depth of LFD

Fig 31.17 **Transverse scan at L3–L4 intervertebral space**

Diagram of scan

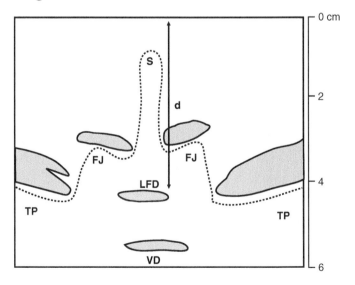

S	Vertebral spine
FJ	Facet joints
TP	Transverse processes
LFD	Ligamentum flavum/dura complex
VD	Ventral dura

Fig 31.18

81

Anatomy of the lumbar plexus

The lumbar plexus is formed by the spinal nerve roots from L1 to L5, and lies within the psoas major compartment. The lumbar plexus passes through and around the fibres of the psoas muscle, forming the femoral nerve (L2,3,4), lumbosacral trunk (L4,5) and obturator nerve (L2,3,4). Additional smaller nerves are also formed, which are the lateral femoral cutaneous (L2,3), iliohypogastric (L1), ilioinguinal (L1) and genitofemoral (L1,2). These smaller nerves exit the psoas compartment and supply the skin over the lateral thigh, lower abdominal wall and groin. The psoas compartment provides a convenient location for blocking the lumbar plexus, and thus providing regional anaesthesia for lower limb surgery.

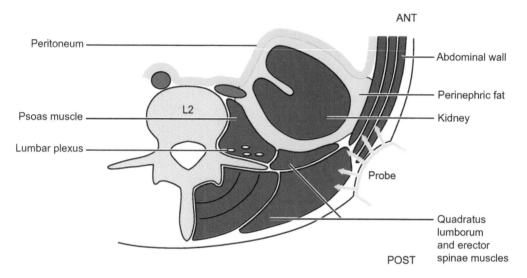

Fig 32.1 **Coronal section at L2 showing psoas major compartment**

Probe placement for lumbar plexus block

Place the patient in a lateral position and apply a curvilinear probe transversely over the lateral aspect of the upper abdominal wall just beneath the costal margin, aiming the probe towards L2.

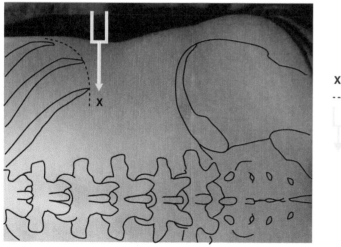

X   Needle entry point
------- Costal margin
    Probe

Fig 32.2 **Probe placement for lumbar plexus block**

Scan of psoas compartment for lumbar plexus block

The bony profile of L2 can be recognized by the reflections from the transverse process and vertebral body. The kidney is relatively 'translucent' on the left side of the scan anterior to L2. The psoas compartment is typically muscle in texture and located between the kidney and the reflection from the transverse process of L2.

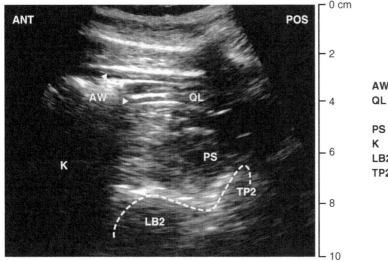

AW Abdominal wall muscles
QL Quadratus lumborum muscle
PS Psoas muscle
K Kidney
LB2 L2 vertebral body
TP2 L2 transverse process

Fig 32.3 **Scan of psoas major compartment at L2 for lumbar plexus block**

Diagram of scan

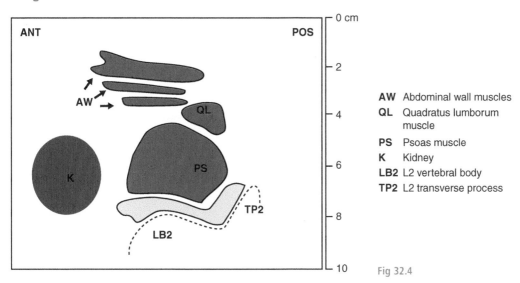

AW Abdominal wall muscles
QL Quadratus lumborum muscle
PS Psoas muscle
K Kidney
LB2 L2 vertebral body
TP2 L2 transverse process

Fig 32.4

Tips and complications Use a curvilinear probe for increased depth of penetration. The lumbar plexus is located in the medio-posterior third of the psoas compartment. The spread of local anaesthetic in the psoas compartment can be monitored by scanning the probe caudally and cephalad to observe levels above and below L2. Perform the technique in plane. Complications include vascular puncture (aorta or inferior vena cava), ureteric puncture, renal puncture and neuraxial blockade.

Juxtamedian (longitudinal) view of the thoracic spine

Ultrasound can be used to examine the thoracic spine in order to help the insertion of thoracic epidural injections and thoracic paravertebral injections. A longitudinal scan in the median plane (midline) is poor because of the angulation and overlap of the vertebral spines. Thus a juxtamedian plane is used which passes through the interspinous gap. Fig. 33.1 shows a median sagittal section through T6 and T7. The juxtamedian ultrasound beam passes from the far side of the vertebral spine, producing reflections at the lamina and base of spine (broken red lines). Where the ultrasound passes between the spines it is reflected from the ligamentum flavum/dorsal dura complex and ventral dura (solid red lines).

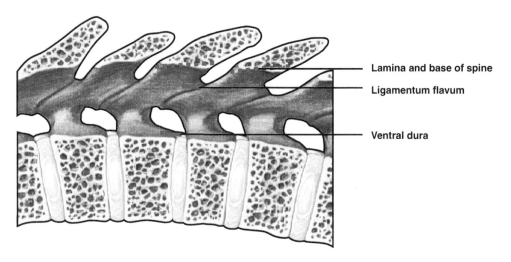

Lamina and base of spine

Ligamentum flavum

Ventral dura

Fig 33.1 **Median section of thoracic spine at T6 and T7**

Probe placement to view thoracic ligamentum flavum

Locate the probe over the median plane initially and then move laterally so that the probe lies over the lamina. Tilt the probe towards the midline to obtain the best view of the ligamentum flavum.

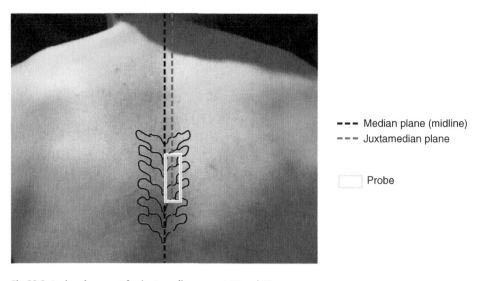

– – – Median plane (midline)

- - - Juxtamedian plane

☐ Probe

Fig 33.2 **Probe placement for juxtamedian scan at T6 and T7**

Juxtamedian scan at T6 and T7

This scan of the thoracic spine shows the positions of the spines and bodies of T6 and T7 (broken yellow lines). Reflections are shown at their bases where the spines meet the laminae. The ultrasound penetrates the interspinous space to give reflections from the ligamentum flavum and ventral dura.

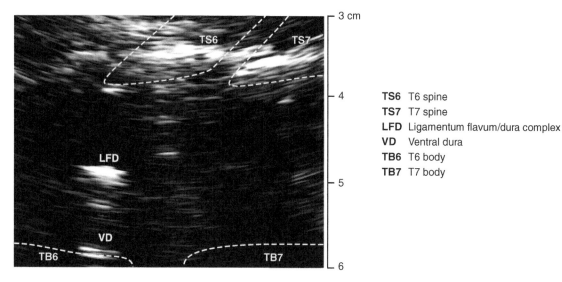

TS6	T6 spine
TS7	T7 spine
LFD	Ligamentum flavum/dura complex
VD	Ventral dura
TB6	T6 body
TB7	T7 body

Fig 33.3 **Juxtamedian scan of thoracic spine at T6 and T7**

Diagram of scan

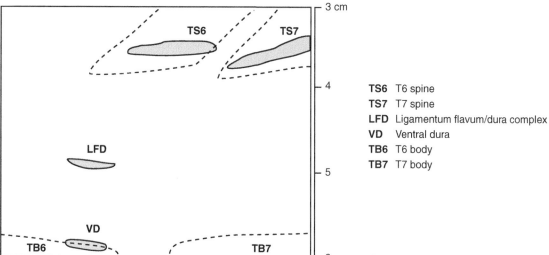

TS6	T6 spine
TS7	T7 spine
LFD	Ligamentum flavum/dura complex
VD	Ventral dura
TB6	T6 body
TB7	T7 body

Fig 33.4

Transverse view of thoracic spine

A transverse view of the thoracic spine can also be used to obtain a view of the ligamentum flavum. As when obtaining the longitudinal view, this is best achieved by placing the centre of the probe over the juxtamedian plane, rather than using the median plane. This is because in the median plane the angulation of the thoracic vertebral spines causes them to overlap and obscure the view of the interspinous space.

The transverse section at T6–T7 shows the parts of the vertebra and the ligamentum flavum which provide reflections in a transverse scan. These are the transverse process (TP), the articular process (AP) and the ligamentum flavum/dura complex (LFD), which highlighted in red.

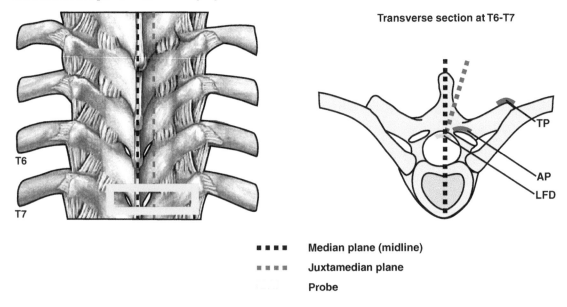

Fig 33.5 **Transverse section of thoracic spine at T6 and T7**

Probe placement for transverse scan of thoracic spine

Start with the probe transversely over the median plane, and then move laterally to centre over the juxtamediam plane with a tilt towards the midline to improve view of the ligamentum flavum. Finally angle in a cephalad direction to optimize the view.

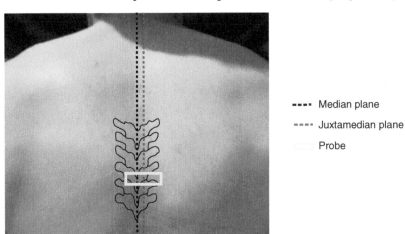

Fig 33.6 **Probe placement for transverse scan at T6 and T7**

Transverse scan at T6–T7

The transverse scan at T6–T7 is centred over the juxtamedian plane, and thus the spine of T6 appears 'off centre'. Reflections are produced by the articular process and transverse process of T7. Note that the transverse process of T7 appears in the same ultrasound plane as the T6 spine, because of the angulation of the thoracic spines. The transverse profile of the thoracic vertebra is outlined in broken yellow (compare with Fig. 33.5).

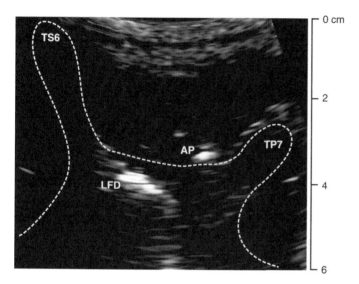

Fig 33.7 Transverse scan at T6 and T7 (centred over juxtamedian plane)

TS6	T6 spine
TP7	T7 transverse process
AP	Articular process
LFD	Ligamentum flavum/dura complex

Diagram of scan

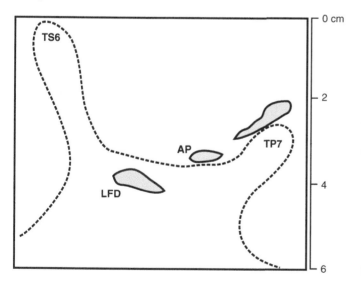

Fig 33.8

TS6	T6 spine
TP7	T7 transverse process
AP	Articular process
LFD	Ligamentum flavum/dura complex

Paravertebral scan through thoracic transverse processes

This is a longitudinal scan which is useful when examining the thoracic paravertebral space (TPVS). The TPVS is the potential space between the costotransverse ligament and the parietal pleura (see *anatomy of the thoracic paravertebral space*). The tips of the transverse processes articulate with the ribs and produce easily recognizable drop-out shadows on scanning in a paravertebral plane (reflecting surfaces highlighted in red).

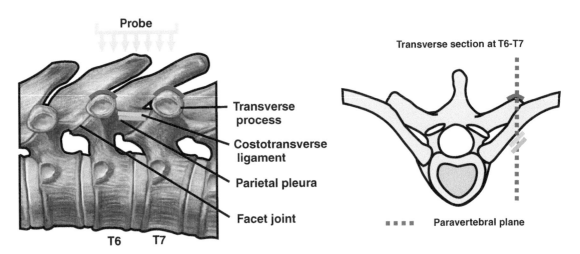

Fig 33.9 **Lateral view of thoracic spine at T6 and T7**

Probe placement for paravertebral scan through thoracic transverse processes

Initially locate the distance of the tips of the transverse processes from the midline, by scanning in a transverse plane. Then rotate the probe through 90 degrees to lie in the paramedian plane of the transverse processes.

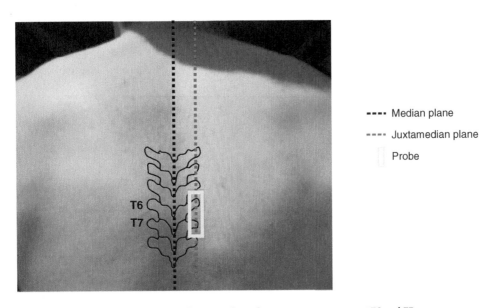

Fig 33.10 **Probe placement for paramedian scan through transverse processes at T6 and T7**

88

Paravertebral scan through transverse processes at T6 and T7

The main landmarks in this scan are the reflections and drop-out shadows from the tips of the transverse processes. The external intercostal muscle and costotransverse ligament lie between the transverse processes. Deep to these layers the pleurae can be recognized by their movement with respiration.

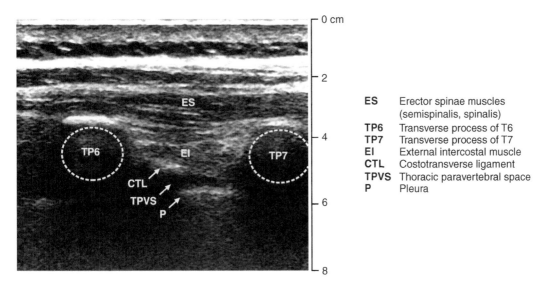

Fig 33.11 Scan in paramedian plane through transverse processes at T6 and T7

ES	Erector spinae muscles (semispinalis, spinalis)
TP6	Transverse process of T6
TP7	Transverse process of T7
EI	External intercostal muscle
CTL	Costotransverse ligament
TPVS	Thoracic paravertebral space
P	Pleura

Diagram of scan

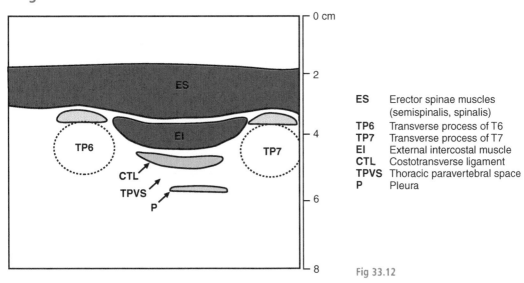

ES	Erector spinae muscles (semispinalis, spinalis)
TP6	Transverse process of T6
TP7	Transverse process of T7
EI	External intercostal muscle
CTL	Costotransverse ligament
TPVS	Thoracic paravertebral space
P	Pleura

Fig 33.12

Anatomy of the thoracic paravertebral space

The thoracic paravertebral space (TPVS) lies adjacent to the veterbral bodies of the thoracic spine and contains the spinal nerves as they emerge from the intervertebral foramina, the anterior division (intercostal nerve), the posterior divison and the rami communicantes. The TPVS connects with the intervertebral foramen medially, and with the potential space between the internal intercostal membrane and the parietal pleura, laterally. This lateral space contains the intercostal nerves.

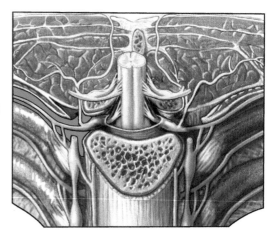

Fig 34.1 **Thoracic paravertebral space (highlighted in blue)**

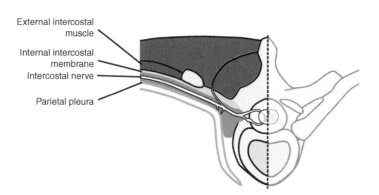

External intercostal muscle
Internal intercostal membrane
Intercostal nerve
Parietal pleura

Fig 34.2 **Boundaries of the TPVS**

Boundaries of the thoracic paravertebral space

The boundaries of the TPVS are illustrated in Fig 34.2. The TPVS is bounded posteriorly by the superior costotransverse ligament and anteriorly by the parietal pleura. The medial boundary is formed by the vertebral body, intervertebral disc and intervertebral foramen. The TPVS at each vertebral level is connected to the level above and below, the caudad limit being the origin of psoas major at T12. The cephalad limit of the TPVS remains undefined.

Probe placement for thoracic paravertebral block

The TPVS may be scanned with a linear or curvilinear probe aligned in the space between two adjacent ribs overlying the transverse process. In this way a needle can be inserted into the TPVS under direct vision using an in-plane technique, thus reducing the possibility of pleural puncture. Use a longitudinal scan initially to identify the plane of the transverse processes (see above).

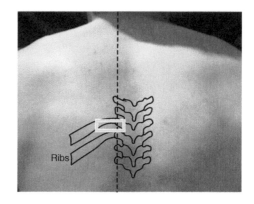

- - - Transverse process plane
☐ Probe

Ribs

Fig 34.3 **Probe placement for thoracic paravertebral block**

Scan of thoracic paravertebral space

The landmarks in this scan are the bony reflection from the transverse process, with its drop-out shadow, and the pleural reflection which moves with respiration.

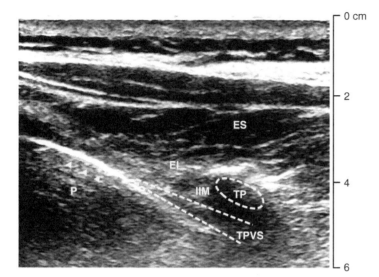

ES	Erector spinae muscles
EI	External intercostal muscles
IIM	Internal intercostal membrane
TP	Transverse process
P	Pleura
TPVS	Thoracic paravertebral space

Fig 34.4 **Scan of the TPVS**

Diagram of scan

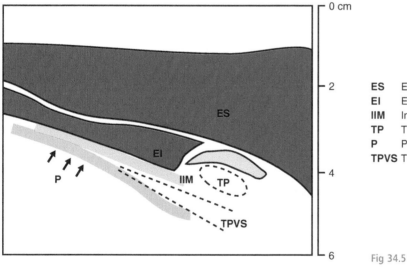

ES	Erector spinae muscles
EI	External intercostal muscles
IIM	Internal intercostal membrane
TP	Transverse process
P	Pleura
TPVS	Thoracic paravertebral space

Fig 34.5

Tips and complications The obvious complication is pneumothorax, due to the proximity of the pleura. Other possibilities are injection into the root canal and epidural or spinal blockade. When performing thoracic paravertebral injection under ultrasound guidance, make sure the needle tip remains visible in plane. Observe the spread of the local anaesthetic into the TPVS as the potential space expands and depresses the parietal pleura.

91

Juxtamedian (longitudinal) view of the cervical spine

Ultrasound can be used to examine the cervical spine in order to help the insertion of cervical epidural injections and cervical facet joint injections. A longitudinal view in the median plane is poor because of the angulation of the vertebral spines. A longitudinal view taken in the juxtamedian plane overcomes this problem and gives a view of the ligamentum flavum and the dorsal dura through the interspinous spaces. These layers are closely related, forming the ligamentum flavum/dorsal dura complex (LFD). In the cervical spine the LFD may be only 2–3 cm from the surface, and the depth of the epidural space is only 1–2 mm.

Fig. 35.1 shows a section through the spinal canal. The broken red lines show where the ultrasound beam strikes the laminae externally on the far side, producing reflections in the scan.

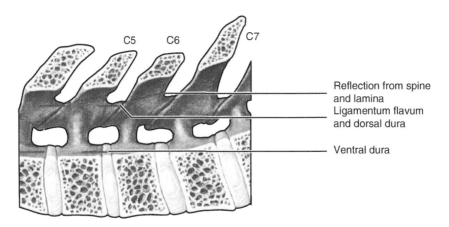

Fig 35.1 **Median longitudinal section of cervical spine at C5–C6**

Probe placement for juxtamedian scan at C5–C6

Locate the probe over the median plane initially and then move laterally into the juxtamedian plane, which lies over the lamina. Tilt the probe towards the midline to obtain the best view of the ligamentum flavum.

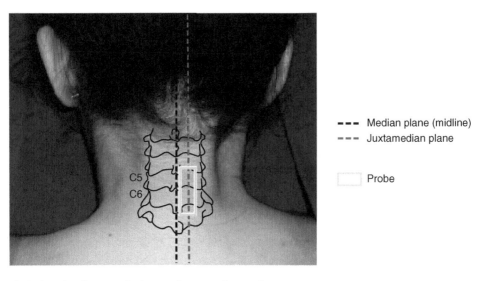

Fig 35.2 **Probe placement for juxtamedian scan of cervical spine at C5–C6**

Juxtamedian scan of cervical spine

In this juxtamedian scan the positions of the cervical vertebral spines and bodies are indicated by the broken yellow outlines. Bright reflections occur at the spine bases and laminae. Between the vertebral spines the ultrasound beam penetrates to give reflections from the composite layer of the ligamentum flavum and dura. Deep to this, reflections from the spinal cord and the ventral dura can be seen.

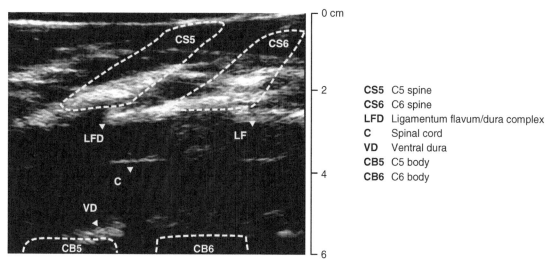

CS5 C5 spine
CS6 C6 spine
LFD Ligamentum flavum/dura complex
C   Spinal cord
VD   Ventral dura
CB5 C5 body
CB6 C6 body

Fig 35.3 **Juxtamedian scan of cervical spine at C5–C6**

Diagram of scan

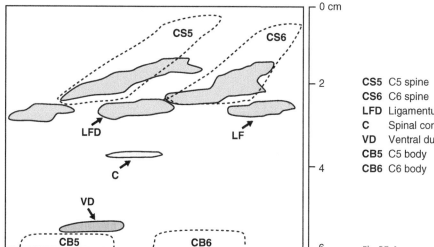

CS5 C5 spine
CS6 C6 spine
LFD Ligamentum flavum/dura complex
C   Spinal cord
VD   Ventral dura
CB5 C5 body
CB6 C6 body

Fig 35.4

Transverse view of cervical spine

A transverse view of the cervical spine can also be used to obtain a view of the ligamentum flavum. This view can be used to measure the depth of the ligamentum flavum for a midline approach to cervical epidural. Interpreting a transverse scan of the cervical spine is aided by identifying the bony features producing reflections in a transverse scan. In Fig. 35.5 the areas reflecting ultrasound are highlighted in red.

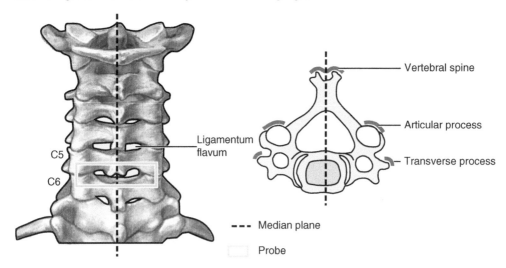

Fig 35.5 **Dorsal view and transverse section of cervical spine at C5–C6**

Probe placement for transverse scan at C5–C6

Place a linear probe transversely over the median plane at C7 and move the probe cephalad, counting the vertebral spines to the intervertebral space between C5 and C6. Then angle the probe in a cephalad direction, in order to obtain the best view of the ligamentum flavum.

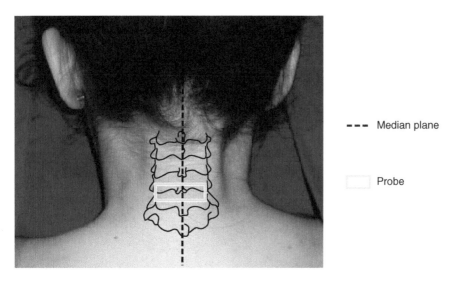

Fig 35.6 **Probe placement for transverse view of cervical spine at C5–C6**

Transverse scan of cervical spine at C5

This transverse scan at C5 shows the bony profile of the cervical vertebra with bright reflections from the spine, articular processes and transverse processes, as illustrated in the cross-section of Fig. 35.5. At this level the dura is closely applied to the ligamentum flavum, the two structures forming a composite layer. Within the spinal canal reflections from the cord and ventral dura are clearly visible.

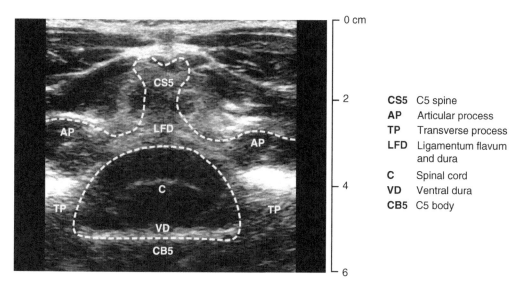

CS5	C5 spine
AP	Articular process
TP	Transverse process
LFD	Ligamentum flavum and dura
C	Spinal cord
VD	Ventral dura
CB5	C5 body

Fig 35.7 **Transverse scan of cervical spine at C5–C6**

Diagram of scan

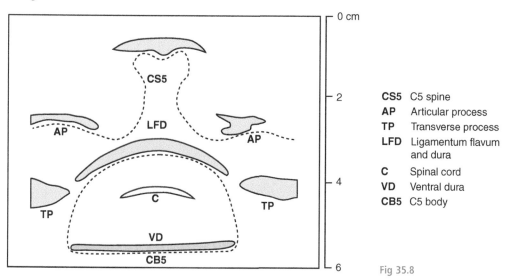

CS5	C5 spine
AP	Articular process
TP	Transverse process
LFD	Ligamentum flavum and dura
C	Spinal cord
VD	Ventral dura
CB5	C5 body

Fig 35.8

Medial branches of the posterior rami of cervical spinal nerves

Each spinal nerve divides into a larger anterior and a smaller posterior ramus after exit from the intervertebral foramen. The posterior rami pass dorsally in close relation to the zygopophyseal processes, to supply the deep muscles of the back (rotatores, multifidus and semispinales). The posterior rami further divide into medial and lateral branches. The medial branches, as well as supplying motor fibres (to the paraspinal muscles), also provide sensory cover to the facet joints and vertebral arch periosteum. These medial branches also supply skin centrally over the spine at their corresponding levels. Medial branch blockade may be successful in treating chronic neck pain symptoms.

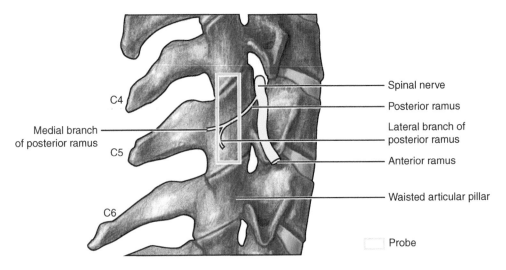

Fig 36.1 **Anatomy of the medial branch of posterior ramus**

Probe placement for block of medial branch of posterior ramus

Initially locate the probe longitudinally over the median plane posteriorly and then move laterally. The probe will pass over the laminae with a flattened overlapping profile (see juxtamedian view, above), to reach the articular pillars, which have a characteristically 'wavy' profile due to the waisted shape of the articular pillar at each level.

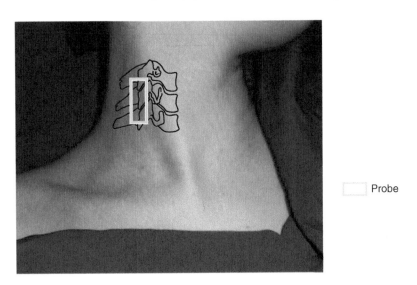

Fig 36.2 **Probe placement for block of the medial branch of posterior ramus**

Scan of C5 articular pillar in cervical spine

The bony profile of the articular pillars is the most recognizable feature of this scan. The waists of the articular pillars create a wavy profile when the probe is aligned along the longitudinal axis of the pillars. The medial branch of the posterior ramus is found at the waist but is not usually visible as a hyperechoic shadow, being too small.

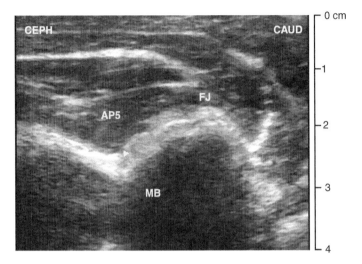

AP5 Waist of C5 articular pillar
FJ Facet joint between C5 and C6
MB Location of medial branch of posterior ramus

Fig 36.3 **Scan of the medial branch of posterior ramus**

Diagram of scan

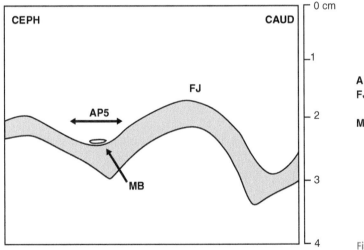

AP5 Waist of C5 articular pillar
FJ Facet joint between C5 and C6
MB Location of medial branch of posterior ramus

Fig 36.4

Tips and complications When locating the probe, scan from the vertebral spines in the median plane to the tips of the transverse processes (posterior border of sternocleidomastoid) in order to confirm probe location over the articular pillar. Complications include intravascular injection and cervical plexus injection.

Anatomy of the sacrum

The sacrum is a triangular bone formed by the fusion of five sacral vertebrae at the base of the spine. Its dorsal surface is marked by a median crest (fused spinous processes), with an intermediate crest (fused articular processes) and lateral crest (fused transverse process tips) on each side. The sacral cornua are bony prominences at the caudal ends of the intermediate crest. The cephalic ends of the lateral crests are also bony prominences (superolateral sacral crests) landmarked superficially by the 'dimples' overlying the posterior superior spines of the ilia. These 'dimples' form the base of an equilateral triangle with the apex at the sacral hiatus, enabling the approximate position of the hiatus to be located when the cornua are not palpable (Fig. 37.1).

The sacrum contains the sacral canal, which is a continuation of the spinal canal containing the termination of the dural sac (S1–S3) and continuation of the epidural space, which terminates at the sacral hiatus with the sacrococcygeal membrane (Fig. 37.2).

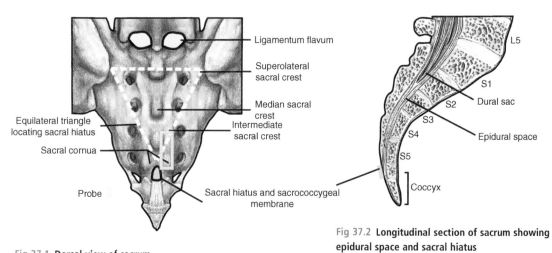

Fig 37.1 **Dorsal view of sacrum**

Fig 37.2 **Longitudinal section of sacrum showing epidural space and sacral hiatus**

Probe placement for longitudinal view of sacral cornua

Use a cuuvilinear probe placed longitudinally over the median crest of the sacrum at the lumbosacral junction, and track the spines of the crest caudally. Move to a paramedian plane laterally below the most caudal spine to find the intermediate crest and the sacral cornu.

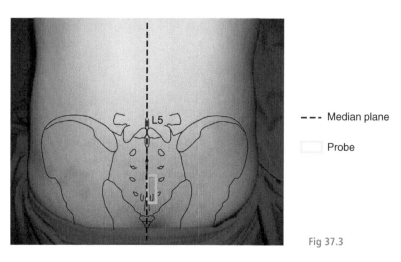

– – – Median plane

☐ Probe

Fig 37.3

Longitudinal scan of intermediate crest and sacral cornua

This paramedian scan at the caudal end of the intermediate crest shows the bright reflections from the peaks of the intermediate crest and the caudal prominence of the sacral cornu (C).

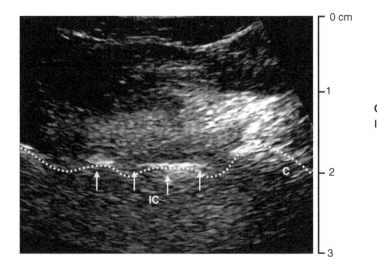

C   Sacral cornu
IC   Profile of intermediate
     sacral crest

Fig 37.4

Diagram of scan

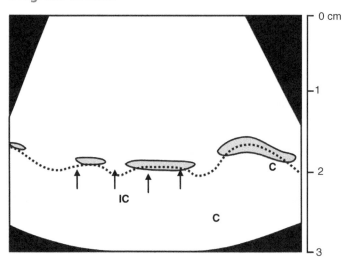

C   Sacral cornu
IC   Profile of intermediate
     sacral crest

Fig 37.5

Transverse view of the sacral cornua

The sacral cornua are often palpable as bony landmarks and can be used to locate the sacral hiatus. The entrance to the hiatus is covered by the sacrococcygeal membrane, which lies between the cornua and extends caudally beyond them.

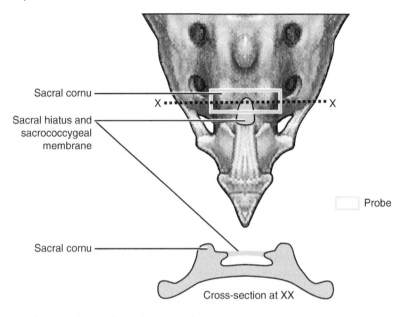

Fig 37.6 **Dorsal view of sacral cornua and sacral hiatus for transverse scan, and cross-section of sacral hiatus**

Probe placement for transverse scan of sacral cornua and sacral hiatus

Use a linear probe placed longitudinally over the median crest of the sacrum and track the spines of the crest caudally. Move in a paramedian plane laterally below the most caudal spine to find the intermediate crest and the sacral cornu. Then rotate the probe through 90 degrees to obtain a transverse view at the level of the sacral cornua.

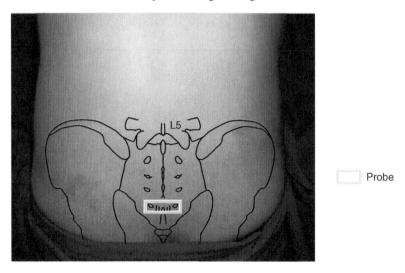

Fig 37.7 **Probe placement for transverse scan of sacral cornua**

Transverse scan of sacral cornua

The transverse scan across the sacral cornua demonstrates their bony profile, with a space between the cornua which is the sacral hiatus. The sacrococcygeal membrane covers the hiatus. A bony reflection deep to the sacral hiatus is the body of S5.

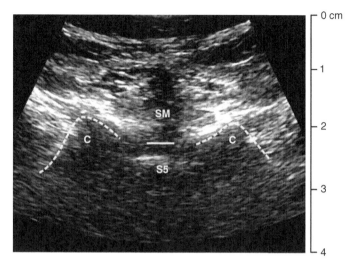

SM Sacrococcygeal membrane
C   Sacral cornua
S5 Body of S5

Fig 37.8 **Transverse scan of sacral cornua**

Diagram of scan

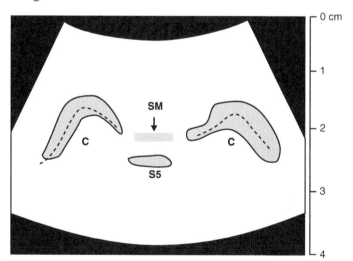

SM Sacrococcygeal membrane
C   Sacral cornua
S5 Body of S5

Fig 37.9

Use of ultrasound in caudal epidural The sacral cornua are the surface landmarks for locating the sacrococcygeal membrane, when performing a caudal epidural injection. These are often palpable, but may not be clearly so in some patients. In such a case use a curvilinear probe to locate the level of the cornua with a longitudinal view of the intermediate crest. Rotate the probe through 90 degrees to obtain a transverse view of the sacral cornua and sacral hiatus. The needle can then be inserted out of plane, and spread of the local anaesthetic can be observed between the sacrococcygeal membrane and the body of S5. In a young child the spread of anaesthetic can often be confirmed in longitudinal view.

Using ultrasound in a lumbar epidural injection

When performing an epidural injection, particularly in a patient with unclear surface anatomy, ultrasound can be used to prescan the patient's spine. This can help to identify:

- The median plane (midline).
- The intervertebral space required.
- Depth of the ligamentum flavum from the skin.
- A suitable entry point and trajectory for the needle.

The procedure used is as follows:

- Identify and mark the midline.
- Identify the lumbosacral junction using a juxtamedian view (see *lumbar spine*) and count the intervertebral spaces cephalad to the space required, maintaining the juxtamedian view.
- Identify the ligamentum flavum/dura complex and note its depth from the skin surface.
- Rotate the probe through 90 degrees to obtain a transverse view of the intervertebral space, and centre the probe over the midline.
- Angle the ultrasound beam slightly in a cephalad direction to obtain the best view of the LFD, and note angle.
- Mark this transverse level. Where this transverse line crosses the midline is the needle entry point.

The prescan defines two perpendicular ultrasound planes, the median (midline) and transverse. The intersection of these planes defines a 'channel' through which the trajectory of the needle should pass (Fig. 38.1).

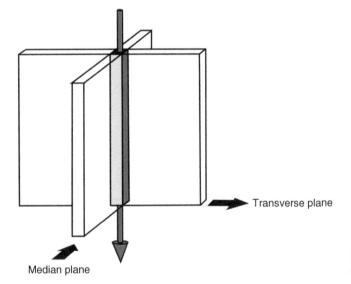

Transverse plane

Median plane

Fig 38.1 **Needle channel as defined by intersection of juxtamedian and transverse scans**

Prescans for lumbar epidural

The prescans are best performed using a curvilinear probe and lower frequencies (2–5 MHz), because of the depth of the LFD and bony landmarks from the surface of the skin. This may reduce the resolution of the scans, but the bony landmarks and ligamentum flavum are usually easily recognized, as shown in *lumbar spine*.

Low-frequency juxtamedian prescan for lumbar epidural

This juxtamedian scan at L2–L3 shows the characteristic 'three-step' reflections produced by the vertebral spines, laminae and LFD. The depth of the LFD from the surface can be obtained from the ultrasound scanner.

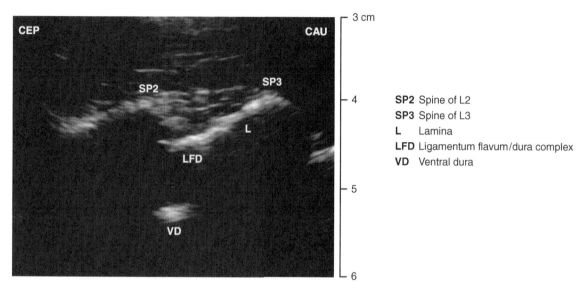

SP2 Spine of L2
SP3 Spine of L3
L　　Lamina
LFD Ligamentum flavum/dura complex
VD　Ventral dura

Fig 38.2 **Juxtamedian prescan for epidural injection**

Low-frequency transverse prescan for lumbar epidural

This transverse prescan shows the reflections from spine, articular processes and transverse processes. The LFD can be seen centrally and its depth can be confirmed.

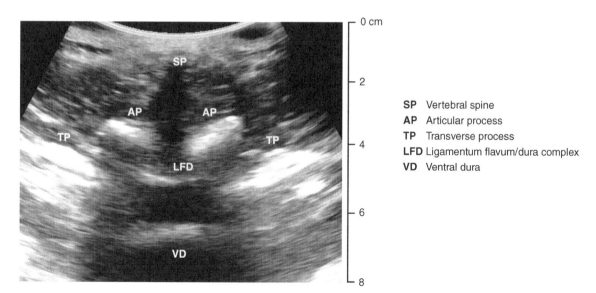

SP　Vertebral spine
AP　Articular process
TP　Transverse process
LFD Ligamentum flavum/dura complex
VD　Ventral dura

Fig 38.3 **Transverse prescan for epidural injection**

103

Anatomy of the greater occipital nerve

The greater occipital nerve (GON) is formed from the medial branch of the posterior ramus of C2, and is a cutaneous nerve supplying sensation to the scalp of the occipital region. It emerges between the transverse process of C2 and the inferior oblique muscle of the head to pierce the semispinalis and trapezius muscles. Subcutaneously the GON lies immediately medial to the occipital artery. Blockade of the GON is used to treat occipital neuralgia.

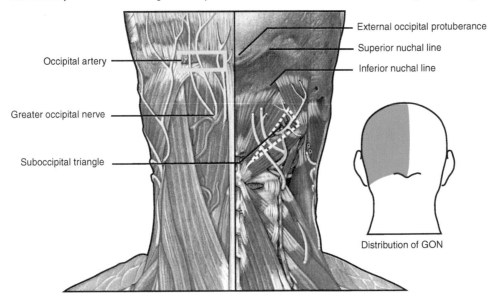

Fig 39.1 **Occipital region and posterior neck (trapezius muscle removed)**

Probe placement for greater occipital nerve block

Palpate and identify the external occipital protruberance (EOP) and superior nuchal line (SNL). The occipital artery can be identified lateral to the EOP. A linear probe is then placed across the space between EOP and the occipital artery.

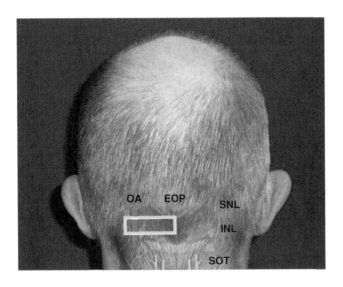

EOP External occipital protuberance
SNL Superior nuchal line
INL Inferior nuchal line
SOT Suboccipital triangle
OA Occipital artery

☐ Probe

Fig 39.2

Scan of greater occipital nerve

The bony boundary of the skull is readily identified, and the main landmark to be identified is the occipital artery superficial to the skull. The occipital nerve lies medial to the artery.

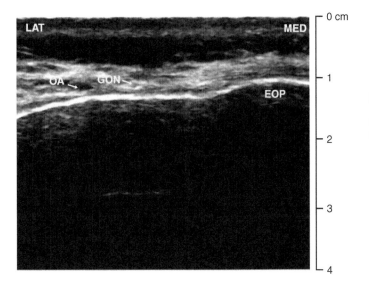

EOP External occipital
     protuberance
GON Greater occipital nerve
OA   Occipital artery

Fig 39.3

Diagram of scan

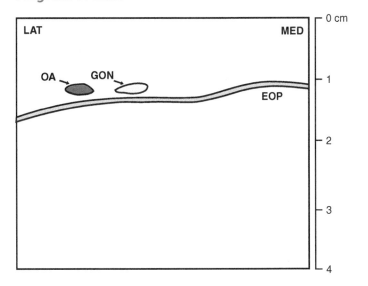

EOP External occipital protuberance
GON Greater occipital nerve
OA   Occipital artery

Fig 39.4

Tips and complications To ensure correct identification of the EOP and superior nuchal line, scan in a saggital plane initially, confirming the 'step' in the bony profile due to the superior nuchal line. Then rotate the probe through 90 degrees. Complications include injection into the suboccipital triangle.

The greater auricular nerve

The greater auricular nerve (GAN) arises from the superficial cervical plexus and contains fibres from C2 and C3 spinal nerves. GAN emerges from the superficial cervical plexus, which lies just deep to the posterior border of the sternocleidomastoid muscle (SCM). It ascends to lie on the surface of SCM, and supplies sensation to the pinna, the skin posterior to the ear, the skin overlying the parotid and the angle of the mandible.

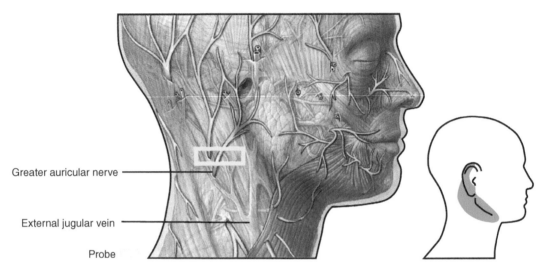

Greater auricular nerve

External jugular vein

Probe

Fig 40.1

Probe placement for greater auricular nerve block

Place a linear probe transversely across SCM at the level of C3 (the level of the hyoid bone), posterior to the external jugular vein (EJV), bridging the space between the EJV and the posterior border of SCM.

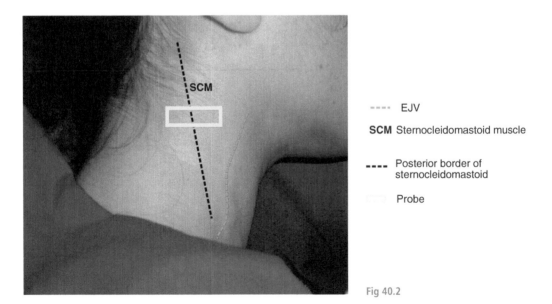

- - - - EJV

SCM Sternocleidomastoid muscle

- - - - Posterior border of sternocleidomastoid

Probe

Fig 40.2

Scan of greater auricular nerve

Identify the posterior edge of SCM, with the internal jugular vein and carotid artery underlying. The GAN may then be visualized subcutaneously, posterior to the EJV.

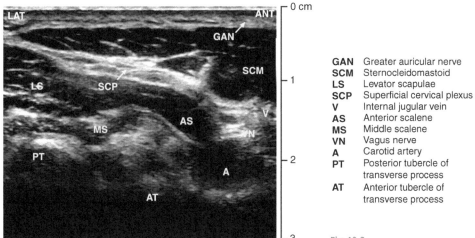

GAN	Greater auricular nerve
SCM	Sternocleidomastoid
LS	Levator scapulae
SCP	Superficial cervical plexus
V	Internal jugular vein
AS	Anterior scalene
MS	Middle scalene
VN	Vagus nerve
A	Carotid artery
PT	Posterior tubercle of transverse process
AT	Anterior tubercle of transverse process

Fig 40.3

Diagram of scan

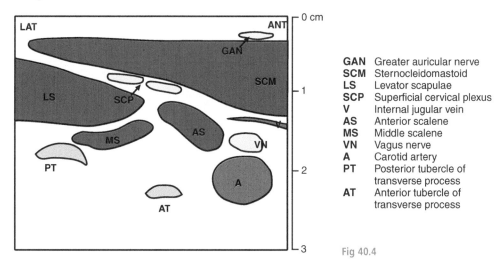

GAN	Greater auricular nerve
SCM	Sternocleidomastoid
LS	Levator scapulae
SCP	Superficial cervical plexus
V	Internal jugular vein
AS	Anterior scalene
MS	Middle scalene
VN	Vagus nerve
A	Carotid artery
PT	Posterior tubercle of transverse process
AT	Anterior tubercle of transverse process

Fig 40.4

Tips and complications This is a small subcutaneous nerve, and use of a nerve stimulator can help needle positioning for lesioning. Keep injection subcutaneous, as complications include injection into structures deep to the sternocleidomastoid muscle and superficial cervical plexus block.

Anatomy of the superficial cervical plexus

The superficial cervical plexus (SCP) is formed by the cutaneous nerves of the cervical plexus, which is derived from the anterior primary rami of C2–C4. The SCP lies just deep to the posterior edge of the sternocleidomastoid muscle at its mid point. This plexus gives rise to the following sensory nerves: the ascending *lesser occipital* and *greater auricular* nerves, the transverse *superficial cervical* nerve and the descending *supraclavicular* nerves.

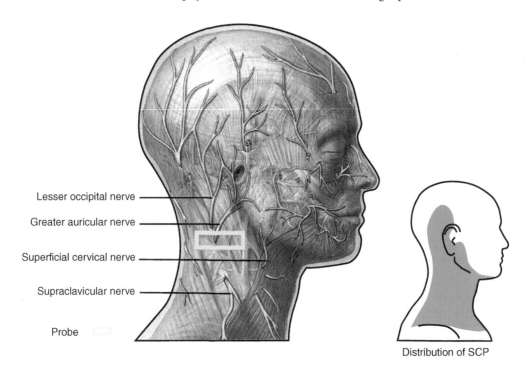

Lesser occipital nerve

Greater auricular nerve

Superficial cervical nerve

Supraclavicular nerve

Probe

Distribution of SCP

Fig 41.1

Probe placement for superficial cervical plexus block

Identify the mid point between the mastoid process and the clavicular head of the sternocleidomastoid muscle. Place a linear probe across the posterior border of sternocleidomastoid muscle at the level of C4 (hyoid bone).

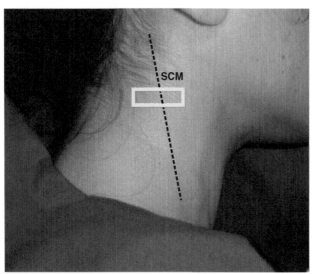

SCM Sternocleidomastoid muscle

- - - - Posterior border of sternocleidomastoid

▭ Probe

Fig 41.2

108

Scan of superficial cervical plexus

Identify the posterior edge of the sternocleidomastoid muscle, with the internal jugular vein and carotid artery underlying. The SCP is seen just deep to the posterior edge of the sternocleidomastoid muscle.

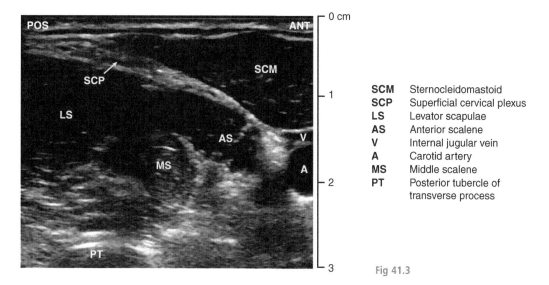

SCM	Sternocleidomastoid
SCP	Superficial cervical plexus
LS	Levator scapulae
AS	Anterior scalene
V	Internal jugular vein
A	Carotid artery
MS	Middle scalene
PT	Posterior tubercle of transverse process

Fig 41.3

Diagram of scan

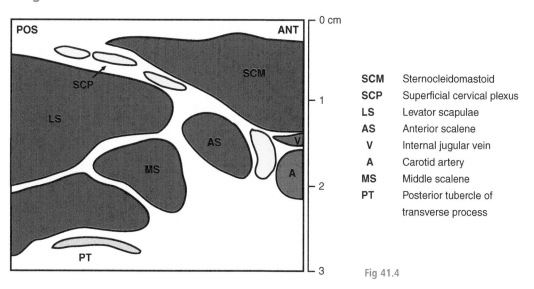

SCM	Sternocleidomastoid
SCP	Superficial cervical plexus
LS	Levator scapulae
AS	Anterior scalene
V	Internal jugular vein
A	Carotid artery
MS	Middle scalene
PT	Posterior tubercle of transverse process

Fig 41.4

Tips and complications Inject in plane and keep the needle tip in view. A deeper injection may produce a cervical plexus block with phrenic nerve palsy, or may puncture jugular and carotid vessels.

Anatomy of the cervical plexus

The spinal nerves emerge from the intervertebral foramina and divide into a large anterior primary ramus (anterior division) and a smaller posterior primary ramus (posterior division). The cervical plexus is formed by the anterior divisions of spinal nerves, C2–C4 (and occasionally C1), which innervate the deep structures of the anterior neck and contribute to the phrenic nerve. Superficial branches from the cervical plexus pass superficially to form the superficial cervical plexus, which provides cutaneous supply for the lateral neck and postauricular area (see *superficial cervical plexus*). The cervical plexus lies in a paravertebral space between the muscles attached to the anterior tubercle of the transverse processes (longus capitis, anterior scalene), and the muscles attached to the posterior tubercle (posterior scalene, middle scalene, levator scapulae). This space is a continuation of the interscalene space.

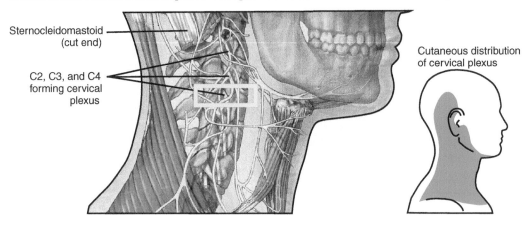

Sternocleidomastoid (cut end)

C2, C3, and C4 forming cervical plexus

Cutaneous distribution of cervical plexus

Fig 42.1

Probe placement for cervical plexus block

Cervical plexus block is a paravertebral block that provides anaesthesia of both superficial and deep structures. It can be used for neck surgery and chronic pain conditions. Place a linear probe transversely across the line connecting the mastoid process to the transverse process of C6 vertebra (Chassaignac's tubercle). C2 lies 2 cm below the mastoid process, C3 is 2 cm below C2, and C4 is 4 cm below C2 on this line. Place the probe transversely across this line on these points to identify the transverse processes of the corresponding vertebrae.

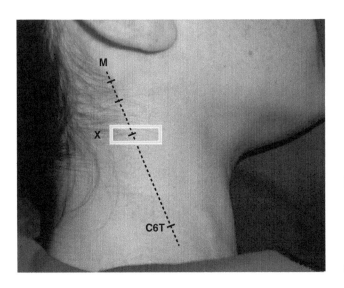

C6T　Chassaignac's tubercle
M　　Mastoid process
X　　Needle entry point

☐　Probe

Fig 42.2

Scan of deep cervical plexus (C4 primary posterior ramus)

In this scan the main landmark to identify is the rounded bony profile of the posterior tubercle of the transverse process. This lies just deep to sternocleidomastoid. The posterior primary ramus can be seen passing posteriorly around the posterior tubercle.

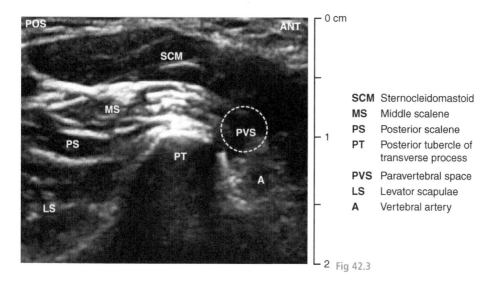

SCM	Sternocleidomastoid
MS	Middle scalene
PS	Posterior scalene
PT	Posterior tubercle of transverse process
PVS	Paravertebral space
LS	Levator scapulae
A	Vertebral artery

Fig 42.3

Diagram of scan

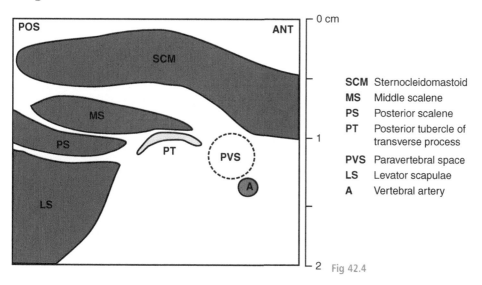

SCM	Sternocleidomastoid
MS	Middle scalene
PS	Posterior scalene
PT	Posterior tubercle of transverse process
PVS	Paravertebral space
LS	Levator scapulae
A	Vertebral artery

Fig 42.4

Tips and complications Use an in-plane technique and approach the paravertebral space from the posterior edge of the probe. Pass the needle tip to contact the posterior tubercle and 'walk' the tip off into the paravertebral space. Inject 2–3 mL of local anaesthetic at each of the required levels.

The needle tip should be visualized at all times. Complications include haematoma, spinal anaesthesia, phrenic nerve block. Avoid bilateral blocks in patients with significant respiratory disease. Use Doppler to identify major vessels, especially the vertebral artery.

Anatomy of the stellate ganglion

The stellate ganglion is the lowest of the cervical sympathetic ganglia. It provides the sympathetic supply to the upper limb, head and neck. It lies in close relation to the transverse process of C7, the dome of the pleura and the vertebral artery. Injection is performed at C6, which helps to avoid these structures.

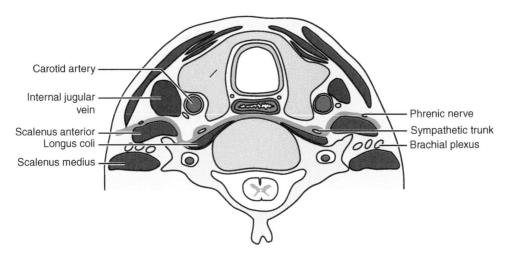

Fig 43.1 **Cross-section of the neck at C6**

Probe placement for stellate ganglion block

Use a linear probe placed over the anterolateral aspect of the neck, overlying the anterior border of the sternocleidomastoid muscle at the level of the cricoid cartilage (C6).

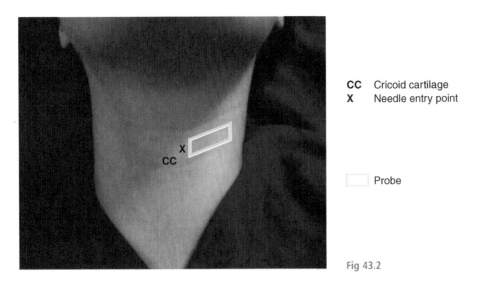

CC Cricoid cartilage
X Needle entry point

☐ Probe

Fig 43.2

Scan of stellate ganglion

The carotid artery is the most obvious landmark in this scan. The trachea is identified over the medial part of the scan, the cricoid cartilage being bright while the lumen of the trachea is dark. The surface of the body and transverse process of C6 is a bright shallow S-shaped curve.

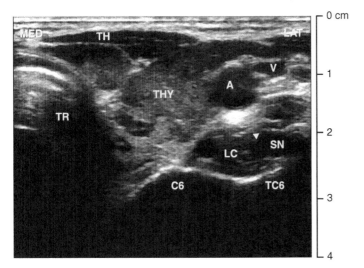

Fig 43.3 **Anterolateral neck at C6**

TH   Thyrohyoid muscle
THY Thyroid
TR   Trachea
A   Carotid artery
V   Internal jugular vein
SN   Sympathetic nerve trunk
LC   Longus coli muscle
C6   Body of C6 vertebra
TC6 Transverse process C6

Diagram of scan

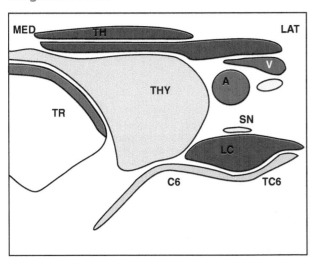

Fig 43.4

TH   Thyrohyoid muscle
THY Thyroid
TR   Trachea
A   Carotid artery
V   Internal jugular vein
SN   Sympathetic nerve trunk
LC   Longus coli muscle
C6   Body of C6 vertebra
TC6 Transverse process C6

Tips and complications Prescan axially above and below the level of the cricoid cartilage, noting the appearance and disappearance of the transverse process of C6 as you move the probe. Mark the position of the probe before proceeding. Insert the needle in plane lateral to the trachea, maintaining a view of the needle tip all the time. Pass medial to the carotid artery until the needle reaches the anterior surface of the longus coli muscle, where the sympathetic nerve trunk is located. Complications are intravascular injection (carotid artery, internal jugular vein, vertebral artery), intrathecal or epidural injection, haematoma.

Anatomy of the subcostal TAP nerves (T7–T10)

The myocutaneous nerves (T7–T10) that supply the upper part of the anterior abdominal wall lie in the fascial plane between the internal oblique and transversus abdominis muscles. This compartment is referred to as the transversus abdominis plane (TAP). These are mixed nerves, supplying the muscles, skin and parietal peritoneum of the upper abdominal wall.

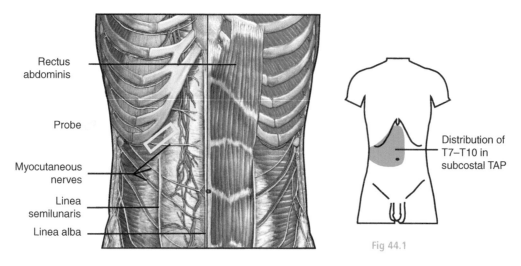

Rectus abdominis

Probe

Myocutaneous nerves

Linea semilunaris

Linea alba

Distribution of T7–T10 in subcostal TAP

Fig 44.1

Probe placement for subcostal TAP block

Start with the probe on the linea alba and move it laterally. The rectus is easily recognized as a single layer of muscle. At the linea semilunaris (lateral border of the rectus sheath) this single layer of muscle divides into three layers: the transversus abdominis (TA), the internal oblique (IO) and the external oblique (EO).

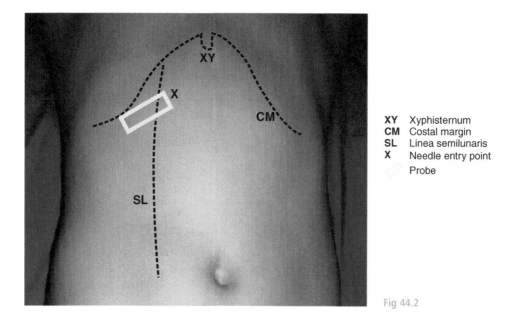

XY   Xyphisternum
CM Costal margin
SL Linea semilunaris
X   Needle entry point
      Probe

Fig 44.2

Scan of subcostal TAP

The three muscle layers of the anterior abdominal wall can be recognized lateral to the edge of the rectus abdominis muscle. The TAP is indicated between the IO and TA muscles.

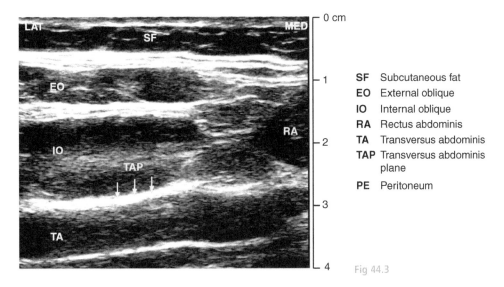

SF	Subcutaneous fat
EO	External oblique
IO	Internal oblique
RA	Rectus abdominis
TA	Transversus abdominis
TAP	Transversus abdominis plane
PE	Peritoneum

Fig 44.3

Diagram of scan

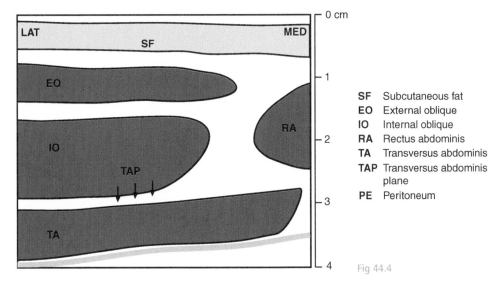

SF	Subcutaneous fat
EO	External oblique
IO	Internal oblique
RA	Rectus abdominis
TA	Transversus abdominis
TAP	Transversus abdominis plane
PE	Peritoneum

Fig 44.4

Tips and complications Use an in-plane technique for both single-shot blocks and catheter insertion. Insert the needle into the TAP and observe the fascial plane opening up as the local anaesthetic is injected. Hydrodissection with saline helps to open the TAP for catheter insertion.

This is relatively free from complications. The needle tip must be visualized at all times, as there is a risk of intraperitoneal injection and bowel perforation.

Anatomy of the lower TAP nerves

The myocutaneous nerves (T10–L1) supply the lower half of the anterior abdominal wall, including the muscle layers and the parietal peritoneum. These nerves lie in a fascial plane referred to as the transversus abdominis plane (TAP), between the internal oblique (IO) and transversus abdominis (TA) muscles.

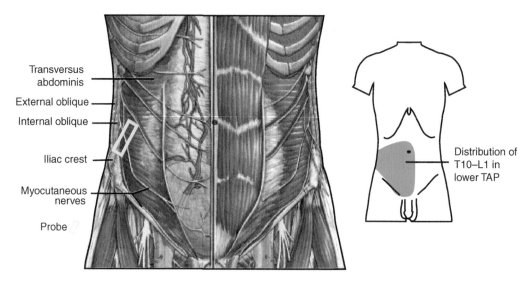

Transversus abdominis

External oblique

Internal oblique

Iliac crest

Myocutaneous nerves

Probe

Distribution of T10–L1 in lower TAP

Fig 45.1 **Anterior abdominal wall (internal oblique, external oblique and rectus muscles removed)**

Probe placement for lower TAP block

Place a linear probe between the iliac crest and the costal margin, over the anterior axillary line, rotating the probe to make an acute angle with the anterior axillary line. This angle improves access for inserting a needle in plane.

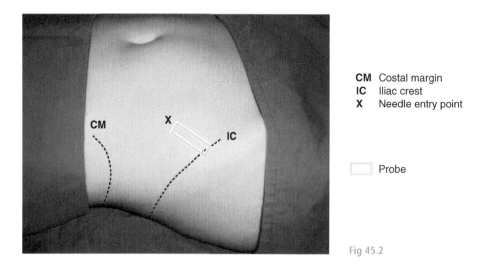

CM

X

IC

CM Costal margin
IC Iliac crest
X Needle entry point

Probe

Fig 45.2

Scan of lower TAP

The iliac crest lies on the left of the scan. Three layers of muscle are visible in the scan deep to the subcutaneous fat. The deepest muscle layer, transversus abdominis, is adjacent to the peritoneum, and bowel can often be recognized beneath this by its peristaltic motion. The TAP lies in the fascial plane between the IO and TA muscles.

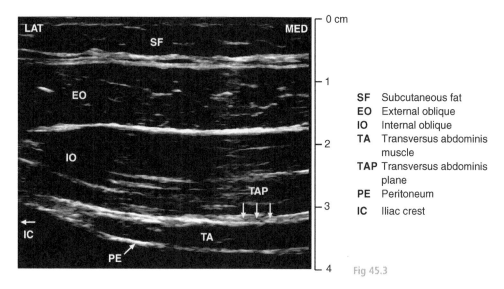

SF	Subcutaneous fat
EO	External oblique
IO	Internal oblique
TA	Transversus abdominis muscle
TAP	Transversus abdominis plane
PE	Peritoneum
IC	Iliac crest

Fig 45.3

Diagram of scan

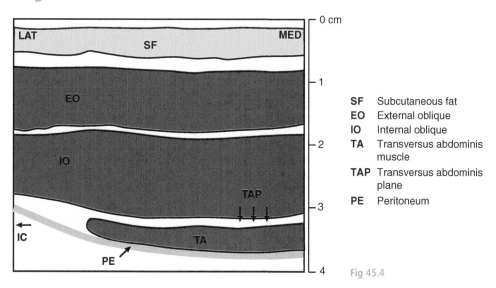

SF	Subcutaneous fat
EO	External oblique
IO	Internal oblique
TA	Transversus abdominis muscle
TAP	Transversus abdominis plane
PE	Peritoneum

Fig 45.4

Tips and complications Use an in-plane technique for both single-shot blocks and catheter insertion. Insert the needle tip into the fascial plane, and on injecting the solution the fascial plane opens up to reveal the potential space between IO and TA muscles. Hydrodissection with saline helps to open the TAP for catheter insertion.

This is relatively free from complications. The needle tip must be visualized at all times, as there is a risk of intraperitoneal injection and bowel perforation.

Anatomy of the Ilioinguinal and iliohypogastric nerves

The ilioinguinal (IIN) and iliohypogastric (IHN) nerves are both terminal branches of the anterior ramus of spinal nerve L1. They are mixed nerves, supplying the internal oblique (IO) and transversus abdominis (TA) muscles as well as the skin over the inguinal and hypogastric areas. These nerves pass towards the inguinal region in the plane between the IO and TA. IIN traverses the inguinal canal to supply the proximal medial thigh and the scrotum or labia majora.

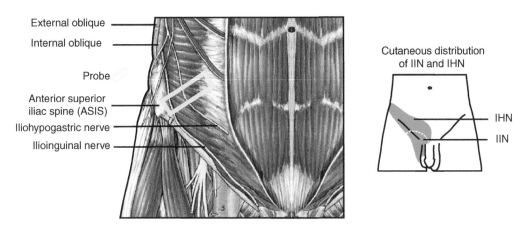

Fig 46.1 **Inguinal region (external oblique and internal oblique muscles removed)**

Probe placement for ilioinguinal and iliohypogastric nerve block

Identify the anterior superior iliac spine (ASIS). Place a linear probe adjacent to the ASIS aligned with the line joining the ASIS to the umbilicus.

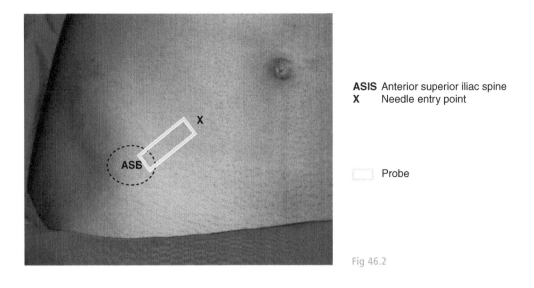

ASIS Anterior superior iliac spine
X Needle entry point

☐ Probe

Fig 46.2

Scan of ilioinguinal and iliohypogastric nerves

The ASIS casts an acoustic shadow at the lateral edge of the scan. The external oblique is only present as an aponeurosis joining with the attachment of the other abdominal wall muscles (IO and TA) to the ASIS. The IIN and IHN are seen in the plane between IO and TA (the 'TAP' plane).

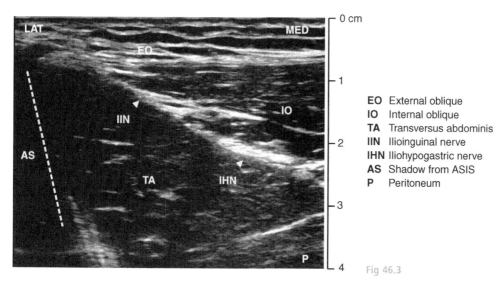

EO External oblique
IO Internal oblique
TA Transversus abdominis
IIN Ilioinguinal nerve
IHN Iliohypogastric nerve
AS Shadow from ASIS
P Peritoneum

Fig 46.3

Diagram of scan

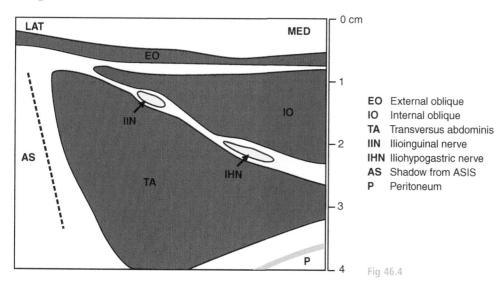

EO External oblique
IO Internal oblique
TA Transversus abdominis
IIN Ilioinguinal nerve
IHN Iliohypogastric nerve
AS Shadow from ASIS
P Peritoneum

Fig 46.4

Tips and complications Needle insertion is performed in plane from the medial aspect of the probe, in order to reduce the risk of peritoneal penetration and bowel perforation.

Anatomy of the rectus sheath nerves (T8–L1)

The rectus sheath nerves are the terminal branches of the myocutaneous nerves (T8–L1) supplying the lower two-thirds of the anterior abdominal wall, including the muscle layers and the parietal peritoneum. They enter the rectus sheath through its lateral border (linea semilunaris) and pass towards the linea alba. Within the rectus sheath the nerves lie between the rectus abdominis muscle and the posterior wall of the sheath, and supply the central abdominal wall.

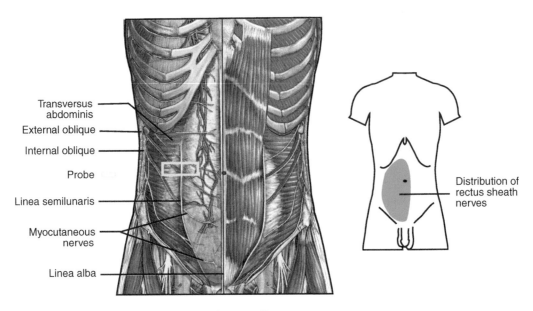

Transversus abdominis
External oblique
Internal oblique
Probe
Linea semilunaris
Myocutaneous nerves
Linea alba

Distribution of rectus sheath nerves

Fig 47.1 **Anterior abdominal wall (rectus muscle removed)**

Probe placement for rectus sheath block

Identify the lateral border of the rectus sheath and place a linear probe transversely across the linear semilunaris at the level of the umbilicus.

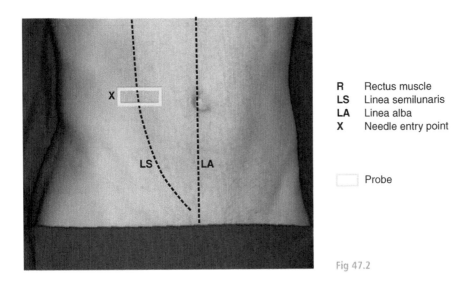

R   Rectus muscle
LS Linea semilunaris
LA Linea alba
X   Needle entry point

☐ Probe

Fig 47.2

Scan of lateral border of rectus sheath

The lateral border of the rectus sheath in the abdominal wall is marked by the transition from the triple layer of muscle (EO, IO, TA) on the left side (lateral) of the scan to the single layer of muscle (RA) on the right (medial). The plane for injection between the RA and the posterior wall of the rectus sheath is indicated as RAP.

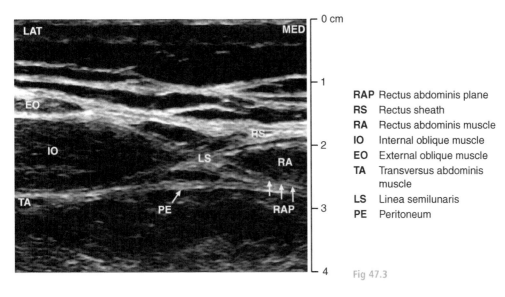

RAP	Rectus abdominis plane
RS	Rectus sheath
RA	Rectus abdominis muscle
IO	Internal oblique muscle
EO	External oblique muscle
TA	Transversus abdominis muscle
LS	Linea semilunaris
PE	Peritoneum

Fig 47.3

Diagram of scan

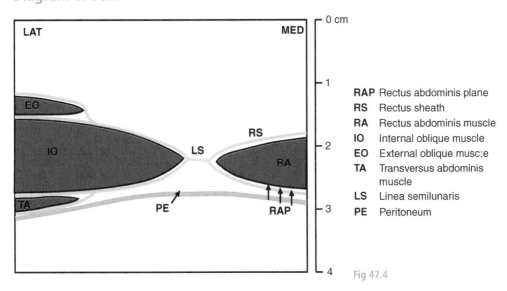

RAP	Rectus abdominis plane
RS	Rectus sheath
RA	Rectus abdominis muscle
IO	Internal oblique muscle
EO	External oblique musc;e
TA	Transversus abdominis muscle
LS	Linea semilunaris
PE	Peritoneum

Fig 47.4

Tips and complications Use an in-plane technique for both single-shot blocks and catheter insertion. Hydrodissection with saline helps to open the rectus sheath plane for catheter insertion. The needle tip must be visualized at all times because of the risk of intraperitoneal injection or bowel puncture.

Anatomy of the genitofemoral nerve

The genitofemoral nerve, GFN (L1,2), is mainly a sensory nerve formed in the lumbar plexus and splitting into femoral (FB) and genital branches (GB). FB supplies the skin over the upper half of the femoral triangle, and GB supplies the anterolateral aspects of the scrotum (or labia majora). Some motor fibres in GB supply the cremaster muscle fibres in the spermatic cord. GFN descends in the psoas compartment to the internal ring, where FB passes under the inguinal ligament in the femoral sheath, while GB enters the spermatic cord where it lies between the cremaster muscle fibres and the internal spermatic fascia. GB exits from the spermatic cord at the pubic tubercle. The ilioinguinal nerve (IIN) also accompanies the spermatic cord (or round ligament in females) in the inguinal canal.

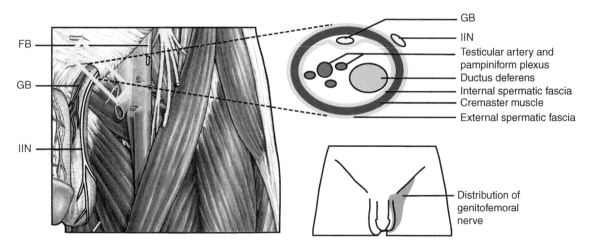

Fig 48.1 **Anatomy of the spermatic cord and distribution of the genitofemoral nerve**

Probe placement for block of genital branch of genitofemoral nerve

Identify the inguinal ligament using the anterior superior iliac spine and pubic tubercle as landmarks. Locate the spermatic cord by palpating it and place a linear probe across the cord just lateral to and above the pubic tubercle.

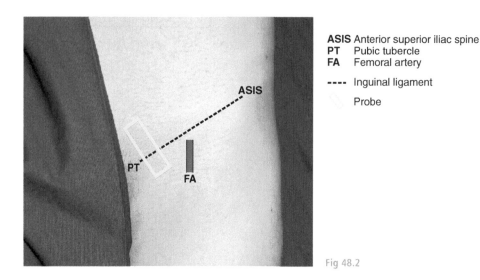

ASIS Anterior superior iliac spine
PT Pubic tubercle
FA Femoral artery

---- Inguinal ligament

Probe

Fig 48.2

Scan of spermatic cord and genitofemoral nerve

The scan of the spermatic cord close to the pubic tubercle shows a characteristic structure with multiple lumens. The lumen with the thickest wall is the ductus deferens, while the testicular artery can be identified using the Doppler setting.

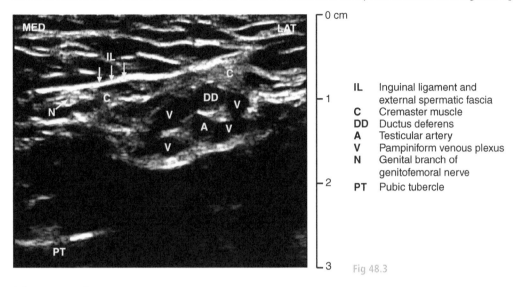

IL	Inguinal ligament and external spermatic fascia
C	Cremaster muscle
DD	Ductus deferens
A	Testicular artery
V	Pampiniform venous plexus
N	Genital branch of genitofemoral nerve
PT	Pubic tubercle

Fig 48.3

Diagram of scan

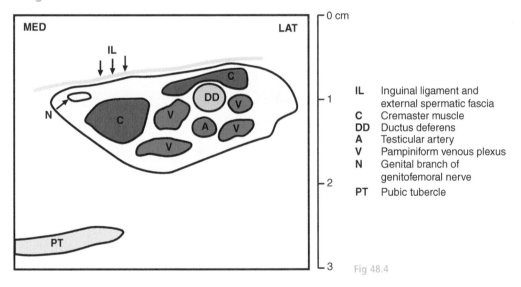

IL	Inguinal ligament and external spermatic fascia
C	Cremaster muscle
DD	Ductus deferens
A	Testicular artery
V	Pampiniform venous plexus
N	Genital branch of genitofemoral nerve
PT	Pubic tubercle

Fig 48.4

Tips and complications For testicular pain inject into the spermatic cord at the pubic tubercle (genital branch). Inject just deep to the external spermatic fascia so that local anaesthetic (LA) passes around the fibres of cremaster muscle between the external and internal spermatic fascial layers. Take care not to traumatize the contents of the cord. Inject small volumes (< 3 mL) in order to avoid compromising the contents of the cord. Also deposit LA around the cord to include the ilioinguinal nerve. Regional block for inguinal hernia requires more lateral injection, over the deep inguinal ring, in order to include both femoral and genital branches of the genitofemoral nerve.

Anatomy of the internal jugular vein

The internal jugular vein (IJV) emerges from the base of the skull through the jugular foramen and descends lying posterolateral to the internal carotid artery and then lateral to the common carotid artery. It joins the subclavian vein to form the brachiocephalic (innominate) vein which drains into the superior vena cava. The IJV, artery and vagus nerve lie together in the carotid sheath, which is under cover of the sternocleidomastoid muscle. Access to this vessel is often required for central venous pressure monitoring and insertion of pulmonary artery catheters.

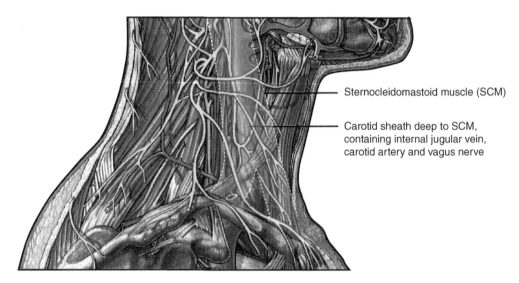

Sternocleidomastoid muscle (SCM)

Carotid sheath deep to SCM, containing internal jugular vein, carotid artery and vagus nerve

Fig 49.1 **Lateral neck (sternocleidomastoid muscle removed)**

Probe placement for cannulation of internal jugular vein

Position the patient supine and turn the head away to the contralateral side. A linear probe is placed across the sternocleidomastoid muscle at approximately the level of C6.

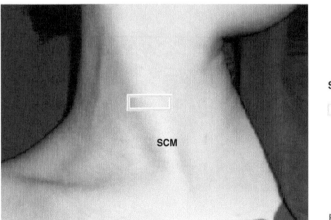

SCM

SCM Sternocleidomastoid

Probe

Fig 49.2

Transverse scan of internal jugular vein

The most visible landmark is the carotid artery. Posterior and superficial to this lies the internal jugular vein which is easily identifiable as it is non-pulsatile, easily compressible and larger in diameter than the artery. These vessels lie closely related to the thyroid, vagus nerve, vertebral artery and trachea.

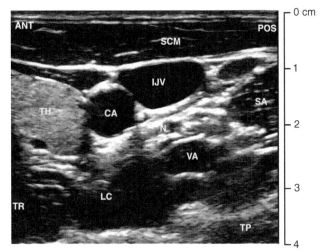

SCM	Sternocleidomastoid muscle
IJV	Internal jugular vein
CA	Carotid artery
TH	Thyroid
N	Vagus nerve
VA	Vertebral artery
SA	Scalenus anterior muscle
LC	Longus coli muscle
TR	Trachea
TP	Transverse process

Fig 49.3

Diagram of scan

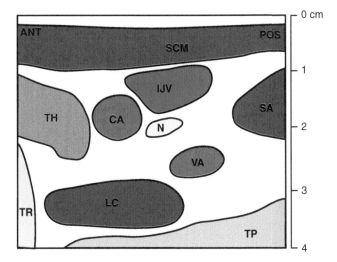

SCM	Sternocleidomastoid muscle
IJV	Internal jugular vein
CA	Carotid artery
TH	Thyroid
N	Vagus nerve
VA	Vertebral artery
SA	Scalenus anterior muscle
LC	Longus coli muscle
TR	Trachea
TP	Transverse process

Fig 49.4

Tips and complications An out-of-plane approach is recommended for the initial needle insertion into the vessel, as the transverse scan visualizes the neighbouring structures, which can be readily traumatized inadvertently. Maintain a shallow approach with the needle. Confirm entry into the vessel by rotating the probe through 90 degrees and using the in-plane view. Turning the head to the contralateral side tightens up the fascial planes around the neck, ensuring the vessels are less mobile underneath. Colour-flow Doppler can be used to differentiate between vessels. Complications include pneumothorax and inadvertent trauma to carotid, subclavian or thyroid vessels. Damage can also occur to the vagus or phrenic nerves.

Anatomy of the femoral vein

The femoral vein lies within the femoral sheath together with the femoral artery. It lies medial to the artery in the sheath. The femoral sheath is located in the femoral triangle, which also contains the femoral nerve. It should be noted that the femoral nerve lies *outside* the sheath. The femoral vein is formed by its tributaries the superficial femoral, the deep femoral and the great saphenous veins which drain the lower limb. The femoral vein exits the femoral triangle by passing deep to the inguinal ligament to become the external iliac vein.

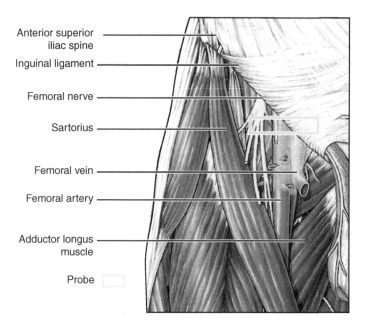

Anterior superior iliac spine
Inguinal ligament
Femoral nerve
Sartorius
Femoral vein
Femoral artery
Adductor longus muscle
Probe

Fig 50.1

Probe placement for femoral venipuncture

Use the borders of the femoral triangle (superior = inguinal ligament, lateral = sartorius muscle, medial = adductor longus), and palpate for the femoral artery. Position a linear probe across the femoral artery pulse.

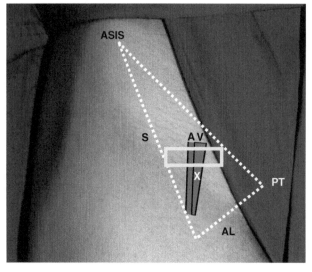

ASIS   Anterior superior iliac spine
S   Sartorius
A   Femoral artery
V   Femoral vein
PT   Pubic tubercle
AL   Adductor longus
X   Needle entry point

        Probe

Fig 50.2

Scan of femoral vein

Use the femoral artery and vein as landmarks. Confirm the identities of the femoral artery with Doppler and the femoral vein by compression with the probe. Note the position of the femoral nerve, lateral to and outside the femoral sheath.

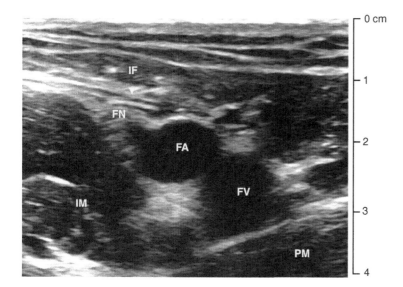

IF   Iliopectineal fascia
FN Femoral nerve
FA Femoral artery
FV Femoral vein
IM Iliopsoas muscle
PM Pectineus muscle

Fig 50.3

Diagram of scan

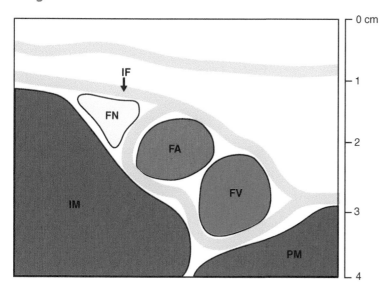

IF   Iliopectineal fascia
FN Femoral nerve
FA Femoral artery
FV Femoral vein
IM Iliopsoas muscle
PM Pectineus muscle

Fig 50.4

Tips and complications Use an out-of-plane approach for needle entry into the vein, as the surrounding anatomy is more clearly displayed with a transverse scan. Confirm needle entry into the vessel by rotating the probe through 90 degrees for an in-plane view. Venipuncture is easier more proximally, just below the inguinal ligament, as the vein tends to pass deep to the artery as the vessels proceed distally into the limb. Complications include arterial puncture and femoral nerve trauma.

Anatomy of the radial artery

The radial artery originates from the bifurcation of the brachial artery just distal to the elbow. It passes distally to the wrist on the radial side of the forearm under cover of brachioradialis. At the wrist the artery becomes superficial, lying over the distal radius and the pronator quadratus muscle. Here it is in close relation to the superficial branch of the radial nerve, which can be damaged inadvertently during arterial puncture. The artery then dives deeply to pass around the lateral side of the carpus, lying over the radial collateral ligament and deep to the tendons of abductor pollicis longus and extensor pollicis brevis. From there it crosses the floor of the anatomical snuff box and enters the dorsum of the hand.

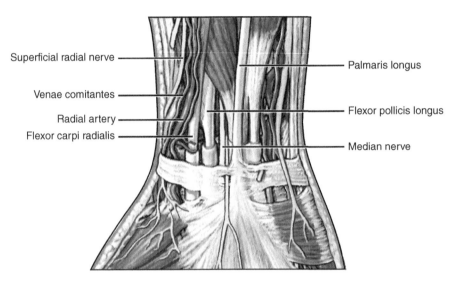

Superficial radial nerve — Palmaris longus
Venae comitantes — Flexor pollicis longus
Radial artery —
Flexor carpi radialis — Median nerve

Fig 51.1

Probe placement for radial artery puncture

Position the patient supine with the arm out and slightly lowered to allow gravity to aid filling. Place a linear probe over the radial pulse on the lateral side of the wrist, proximal to the wrist crease.

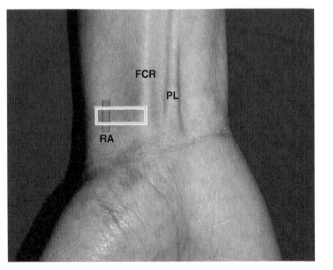

RA Radial artery
FCR Flexor carpi radialis
PL Palmaris longus

☐ Probe

Fig 51.2

Scan of radial artery

There is no difficulty in identifying the radial artery in the scan, but confirm its identity using Doppler.

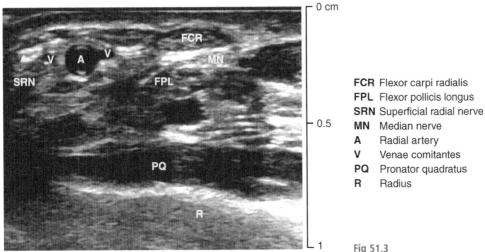

FCR	Flexor carpi radialis
FPL	Flexor pollicis longus
SRN	Superficial radial nerve
MN	Median nerve
A	Radial artery
V	Venae comitantes
PQ	Pronator quadratus
R	Radius

Fig 51.3

Diagram of scan

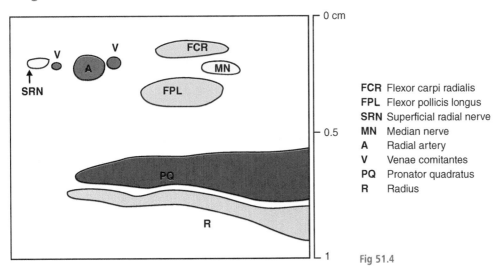

FCR	Flexor carpi radialis
FPL	Flexor pollicis longus
SRN	Superficial radial nerve
MN	Median nerve
A	Radial artery
V	Venae comitantes
PQ	Pronator quadratus
R	Radius

Fig 51.4

Tips and complications Select a site proximal to the wrist crease to avoid the origins of palmar branches of the artery. Check for collateral circulation of the hand. Allen's test is not a satisfactory test of the integrity of the distal and proximal palmar arch circulations. Pulse oximetry may be used to check integrity. Scan the artery transversely initially to identify the local anatomy and track the artery proximally and distally. The radial artery is easily identified in transverse view but may be lost in a longitudinal scan since it only has a small diameter ($< 5 \, mm$) at the wrist. Confirm the identity of the artery using Doppler. Use a shallow approach (< 30 degrees) with the needle in plane.

Complications of arterial puncture include haematoma, shearing of the arterial intima, damage to the superficial radial nerve and thrombus formation.

Anatomy of the subclavian vein

The subclavian veins are tributaries of the innominate (brachiocephalic) veins which drain into the right side of the heart via the superior vena cava. The subclavian vein and artery are formed from the axillary vessels and pass medially under the clavicle, across the upper surface of the first rib. The subclavian vein is medial to the artery at this stage. A useful surface landmark is the deltopectoral triangle (the narrow triangular groove between deltoid, pectoralis major and the clavicle), which overlies the vessels as they pass beneath the clavicle and over the first rib. This is a convenient location for cannulation of the vein, since it is superficial in this area.

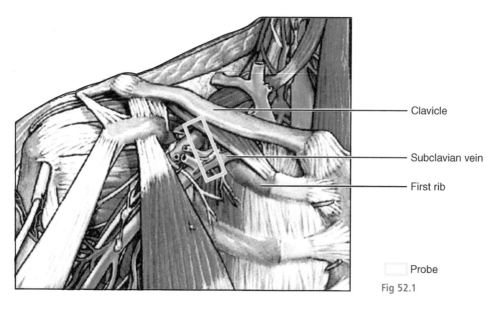

Clavicle

Subclavian vein

First rib

▢ Probe

Fig 52.1

Probe placement for cannulation of subclavian vein

Position the patient supine and head down so as to allow the subclavian vein to fill. Place a linear probe at the mid point of the clavicle across the base of the deltopectoral triangle. It may be possible to palpate the subclavian artery at this point to confirm its location.

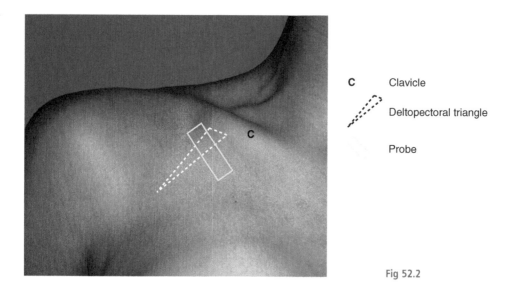

C   Clavicle

Deltopectoral triangle

Probe

Fig 52.2

Scan of subclavian vein

The subclavian artery is easily identifiable, being pulsatile. Confirm its identity with Doppler. In comparison, the subclavian vein is non-pulsatile, compressible and of greater diameter.

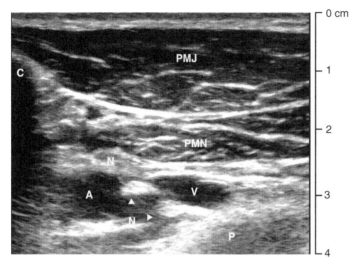

PMJ	Pectoralis major muscle
PMN	Pectoralis minor muscle
C	Clavicle
A	Subclavian artery
V	Subclavian vein
N	Brachial plexus
P	Pleura

Fig 52.3

Diagram of scan

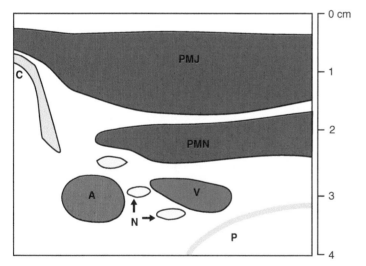

PMJ	Pectoralis major muscle
PMN	Pectoralis minor muscle
C	Clavicle
A	Subclavian artery
V	Subclavian vein
N	Brachial plexus
P	Pleura

Fig 52.4

Tips and complications Use an out-of-plane approach initially, as the transverse scan displays more of the surrounding anatomy. Maintain an angle of approximately 30 degrees for needle entry and vein puncture. Then rotate through 90 degrees for an in-plane view of the needle when entering the vein and to confirm needle placement. Complications include subclavian artery puncture, pneumothorax and haemothorax.